THE CASE OF TERRI SCHIAVO ⠃

The Case of Terri Schiavo ::

Ethics, Politics, and Death in the 21st Century

Edited by

Kenneth W. Goodman

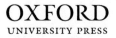

OXFORD
UNIVERSITY PRESS

2010

OXFORD
UNIVERSITY PRESS

Oxford University Press, Inc., publishes works that further
Oxford University's objective of excellence
in research, scholarship, and education.

Oxford New York
Auckland Cape Town Dar es Salaam Hong Kong Karachi
Kuala Lumpur Madrid Melbourne Mexico City Nairobi
New Delhi Shanghai Taipei Toronto

With offices in
Argentina Austria Brazil Chile Czech Republic France Greece
Guatemala Hungary Italy Japan Poland Portugal Singapore
South Korea Switzerland Thailand Turkey Ukraine Vietnam

Copyright © 2010 by Oxford University Press, Inc.

Published by Oxford University Press, Inc.
198 Madison Avenue, New York, New York 10016
www.oup.com

Oxford is a registered trademark of Oxford University Press.

Library of Congress Cataloging-in-Publication Data
The case of Terri Schiavo : ethics, politics, and death in the 21st century /
edited by Kenneth W. Goodman.
    p. ; cm.
Includes bibliographical references and index.
ISBN 978-0-19-539908-0
1. Schiavo, Terri, 1963–2005.   2. Right to die—Moral and ethical aspects—United
States—Case studies.   3. Terminal care—Moral and ethical aspects—United States—Case
studies.   4. Medical ethics—United States—Case studies.   5. Coma—Patients—United
States—Biography.   I. Goodman, Kenneth W., 1954–
[DNLM: 1. Schiavo, Terri, 1963–2005.   2. Euthanasia, Passive—ethics—United
States.   3. Right to Die—ethics—United States.   4. Bioethics—United States.
5. Legislation as Topic—United States.   6. Persistent Vegetative State—United States.
WB 33 AA1 C337 2009]
R726.C358 2009
179.7—dc22

2009010330

Printed in the United States of America
on acid-free paper

PREFACE ⠸

The case of Theresa Schiavo is a watershed in bioethics, U.S. politics, jurisprudence, and health policy. It became clear early on that not only was the case extraordinary, but it had a rare power: a power to anger, to confound, to ennoble.

In assembling the team of contributors to this volume, the goal was to identify leading authorities in the various disciplines that bore on the case. As it developed, several of them were directly involved in the case. They are frank, and their arguments are as forceful as any in contemporary bioethics. There are disagreements herein, and the project is richer for it. Even those not directly involved in the case lived it, and throughout the book one should get the sense of passionate argument tempered by scholarly expertise. The "bioethics community" itself receives reasoned lumps. While books by other key players—husband, parents, lawyers—have appeared, it is necessary to produce a volume to inform and stimulate students as well as professors, patients and clinicians, voters and representatives.

The result, one hopes, is a collection that provides an exciting and comprehensive overview and analysis of key aspects of the case.

The case was exciting. It also became clear early on that it was hard to follow. Schiavo I, Schiavo II ... Schiavo n, with a tangle of suits and appeals and rulings: a mire without precedent. To try to keep it all straight, we began listing and annotating events in a Web-based timeline. Key rulings could then be accompanied by copies of the associated bills, reports, and court opinions. We added a bibliography, a list of links, etc. It was, in many respects, precisely what the World Wide Web is most useful for. The Timeline[1] would have been an uninterpreted flood of dates if not for the legal expertise and supererogatory efforts of Prof. Kathy Cerminara of Nova Southeastern University's Shepard Broad Law Center. Her expertise, shaped by work on the standard reference *The Right to Die*,[2] has also been invaluable at several points in the preparation of this volume. It has been a delightful surprise that the Timeline has itself come to be recognized as a reputable, if not authoritative, resource on the case.

Readers will use the Timeline most profitably by consulting it in conjunction with the chapters here. In cases where it seems particularly apt, notes to the chapters include reminders of documents' availability on the Web.

This book owes much to many. My dear Jacqueline Schneider, an elder law attorney, spent countless hours assisting with the volume's preparation and editing, evincing grace and patience, the latter of which was sorely tried on several occasions. University of Miami Ethics Programs Administrator Gary Dunbar has done superheroic work, as usual, in helping to pull the many pieces together.

Author Ron Cranford, a major figure in bioethics for a quarter-century, died during the preparation of this volume.[3] The chapter here is his last scholarly effort. Special thanks are due to Kristin Cranford, his daughter, Candy Cranford, his wife, and Joanne Roberts, a close friend and scholarly collaborator, for quiet and dignified efforts to polish his manuscript and make it ready for publication during a very difficult time. A statement prepared by family members noted that "Dr. Cranford will long be recognized as a forerunner in advocating that individuals establish health care directives, the right of the patient to make informed health decisions and the right of family members to carry out the expressed wishes of the patient. Those rights he so passionately advocated for others, he demonstrated in his own life and his passing."

Thanks are due the Florida Bioethics Network and its board and members for providing a nonpartisan platform for airing a variety of ideas, some of them controversial. (Several passages of my chapter here first appeared in *Florida Bioethics*, the FBN's newsletter.) Colleagues from universities across Florida were in regular touch during the most heated seasons of the case, and the result is a collegial network dedicated to improving ethics education. FBN Board Member Robin N. Fiore, a contributor to this volume, has been a wise and generous collaborator, and her patient insights and editing advice have improved the volume in ways too numerous to count.

We are indebted to Peter Ohlin at Oxford University Press for his insight and encouragement. Anita Cava and Jacqueline Goodman helped keep the coast clear when necessary. Allison Goodman continued to ask superb questions and learned how to juggle many complex ideas, and balls, during the preparation of this book.

University of Miami students of philosophy, medicine, religious studies, law, and other disciplines have for years constituted precious audiences for testing both arguments and intuitions as the case unfolded, and since. They were a constant reminder of the primacy of education in politics, policy, and ethics.

Kenneth W. Goodman
Miami
January 2009

NOTES

1. Cerminara, K.L., and Goodman, K.W. Key events in the case of Theresa Marie Schiavo. Available at http://www.miami.edu/ethics/schiavo/schiavo_timeline.html.
2. Meisel, A., and Cerminara, K.L. *The Right to Die: The Law of End-of-Life Decisionmaking.* New York: Aspen, 3rd ed., 2004.
3. Pearce, J. Ronald E. Cranford, 65, an expert on coma, is dead. *The New York Times,* June 3, 2006, p. A14.

Contents ⠿

Contributors   *xi*

1. Terri Schiavo and the Culture Wars: Ethics vs. Politics   *1*
   Kenneth W. Goodman

2. At Theresa Schiavo's Bedside: A Guardian's Role
   and Reflections   *39*
   Jay Wolfson

3. *Schiavo*, Privacy, and the Interests of Law   *50*
   Daniel N. Robinson

4. The *Schiavo* Maelstrom's Potential Impact on the Law of
   End-of-Life Decision Making   *78*
   Kathy L. Cerminara

5. The Continuing Assault on Personal Autonomy in the Wake of
   the Schiavo Case   *101*
   Jon B. Eisenberg

6. A Common Uniqueness: Medical Facts in the Schiavo Case   *112*
   Ronald E. Cranford

7. Crossing the Borderlands at Nightfall: New Issues in Moral
   Philosophy and Faith at the End of Life   *137*
   Laurie Zoloth

8. Disability Rights and Wrongs in the Terri Schiavo Case   *158*
   Lawrence J. Nelson

9. Framing Terri Schiavo: Gender, Disability, and Fetal Protection   *191*
   Robin N. Fiore

10. Terri Schiavo and Televised News: Fact or Fiction?   *210*
    Robert M. Walker
    Jay Black

    Appendix: Timeline of Key Events in the Case of Theresa Marie Schiavo   *225*

    Index   *255*

CONTRIBUTORS ⁑

Jay Black, Ph.D., has retired as Poynter Jamison Chair in Media Ethics and Press Policy, Emeritus, at the University of South Florida in St. Petersburg. For 22 years he was editor of the *Journal of Mass Media Ethics.* He has authored 10 editions of media and society and media ethics texts and written or presented some 500 papers/seminars/addresses, most of them on applied professional ethics.

Kathy L. Cerminara, J.D., LL.M., J.S.D., Professor of Law at the Nova Southeastern University Shepard Broad Law Center, is co-author of the third edition of the treatise, *The Right to Die: The Law of End-of-Life Decisionmaking* (Aspen). At NSU's law school, she teaches Torts, Civil Procedure, and health-law–related courses. She also created, was the initial director of, and teaches in the online Master of Science in Health Law program for non-lawyers. She has written several articles in legal and legal-medical journals on both end-of-life decision making and patients' rights in managed care.

Ronald E. Cranford, M.D., was a Senior Physician in Neurology at Hennepin County Medical Center in Minneapolis, a Professor of Neurology at the University of Minnesota, and a Faculty Associate at the University of Minnesota's Center for Bioethics. By the time of his death in June 2006, he was the author of more than 90 articles in neurology, including brain death, coma, and vegetative states; bioethics; and public policy. In addition to examining Ms. Schiavo (in 2002, before the case became widely known), he consulted on several other key end-of-life cases.

Jon B. Eisenberg, J.D., was one of the attorneys on Michael Schiavo's side in the Terri Schiavo case and represented a nationwide group of bioethicists as *amici curiae* in the case. He has litigated in appellate courts on a variety of civil rights and business issues, including free speech, the right to die, reproductive choice, mediation, ethics, and corporate fraud. He is with the law firm of Eisenberg & Hancock LLP and teaches appellate procedure at University of California Hastings Law School in San Francisco.

Robin N. Fiore, Ph.D., is Adelaide R. Snyder Professor of Ethics and Associate Professor of Philosophy at Florida Atlantic University in Boca Raton; she also holds an appointment as Voluntary Associate Professor of Medicine in the Department of Medicine at the University of Miami Miller School of Medicine. Dr. Fiore is a Visiting Scholar at the Center for Women Policy Studies in Washington. D.C. Her publications include articles on informed consent, clinical professionalism, conflicts of interest in research, and topics in women's bioethics.

Kenneth W. Goodman, Ph.D., is a Professor of Medicine and jointly of Philosophy at the University of Miami, where he directs the Bioethics Program and co-directs the Ethics Programs. He also is director of the Florida Bioethics Network. He is the author of *Ethics and Evidence-Based Medicine: Fallibility and Responsibility in Clinical Science* (Cambridge University Press), co-author of *Ethics and Information Technology: A Case-Based Approach to a Health Care System in Transition* (Springer), and has written articles in bioethics, information technology, and the philosophy of science.

Lawrence J. Nelson, Ph.D., J.D., is a Senior Lecturer in Philosophy at Santa Clara University in Santa Clara, California. He is Faculty Scholar in the Markkula Center for Applied Ethics. He primarily teaches undergraduate courses in bioethics, law and ethics, ethical theory, and feminist ethics. He practiced law from 1981 to 1986 with a firm in San Francisco and provided bioethics consultation and education as an independent practitioner from 1986 to 1996. Dr. Nelson has published articles on ethics, law, and health care, including a recent law review article on constitutional personhood and abortion, and served as a bioethics consultant to projects of the National Institutes of Health, the Hastings Center, and the American Thoracic Society.

Daniel N. Robinson, Ph.D., is a member of the Oxford University Philosophy faculty and is Distinguished Professor, Emeritus, Georgetown University, on whose faculty he served for 30 years. Author and editor of more than 40 volumes, Professor Robinson's scholarship covers an unusually wide range of disciplines, including the brain sciences, philosophy and history of science, moral philosophy, philosophy of law, philosophy of mind, and intellectual history. In 2001 he received the Lifetime Achievement Award from the Division of the History of Psychology of the American Psychological Association and, in the same year, the Distinguished Contribution Award from the APA's Division of Theoretical and Philosophical Psychology. He has served as consultant to a number of governmental and private organizations, including the National Science Foundation, the National Institutes of Health, and the Department of Health and Human Services. Columbia University Press published his *Consciousness and Mental Life* in 2008.

Robert M. Walker, M.D., is Director of the Division of Ethics, Humanities, & Palliative Medicine at the University of South Florida College of Medicine, Tampa, where he is an Associate Professor in the Department of Internal Medicine. He has leadership roles at several Tampa-area health care organizations. Dr. Walker is the author of a number of influential papers on end-of-life care, clinical futility, and other topics.

Jay Wolfson, Dr.P.H., J.D., is the Distinguished Service Professor of Public Health and Medicine at the University of South Florida in Tampa. He is Associate Vice President for Health Law, Policy and Safety and Director of the Suncoast Center for Patient Safety. In 2003, he was appointed as Theresa Schiavo's guardian ad litem, reporting to the governor and the courts. He also serves as Special Counsel to the Florida Office of the Attorney General on fraud and abuse in the dialysis industry. He conducts research, writes, and speaks about health care law, ethics, policy, and finance.

Laurie Zoloth, Ph.D., is Director of the Center for Bioethics, Science and Society and Professor of Medical Ethics and Humanities at Northwestern University, Feinberg School of Medicine, and Professor of Religion and a member of the Jewish Studies faculty at Northwestern University, Weinberg College of Arts and Science. She directs bioethics at the Center for Genetic Medicine, the Center for Regenerative Medicine, and the Institute for Nanotechnology. From 1995 to 2003, she was Professor of Ethics and Director of the Program in Jewish Studies at San Francisco State University. In 2001, she was the President of the American Society for Bioethics and Humanities as well as serving on its founding board for two terms.

1 ::

Terri Schiavo and the Culture Wars: Ethics vs. Politics

Kenneth W. Goodman

:: From Family Tragedy to Political Drama

It is the most extraordinary end-of-life case, ever.

By the time Terri Schiavo died on March 31, 2005, at Hospice of the Florida Suncoast in Clearwater, the nation—indeed the world—had eavesdropped on a family conflict with no equal, had witnessed unprecedented legislative machinations in the state capital and in Washington, and had seen dozens of courts hear and rule on scores of motions and pleadings that addressed cornerstone issues in end-of-life care: What are the powers of guardians and other surrogates? How much evidence is needed before their requests or refusals are honored? What is the role of government in bedside medical decisions? How should "disability" be defined? Are artificial nutrition and hydration like or unlike other forms of treatment?

Then, when politics intervened in the kind of case familiar to many hospital ethics committees, the Terri Schiavo story turned from tragedy to farce. At one point, the Congress of the United States of America subpoenaed the permanently unconscious Ms. Schiavo to appear and testify. It was a riot of kooky views and political vehemence.

The brightest light in the ultra-heated debate was that ordinary people talked about it with their family and friends. They talked about life, cognition, and death. They talked about what they value in being alive. They talked about advance-care planning, including living wills. In survey after survey, ordinary people said they would not want to live like Terri Schiavo.

And who would? That some *said* they would seemed to make sense only as an act of keeping faith with Culture War comrades. As Terri Schiavo became a heroine of rightist resurgence in post-New Deal America, it became disloyal to suggest that you didn't desire a life of permanent unconsciousness. The dominant value here was that of "vitalism," a view that holds that all human life (even humans who have no mental life, no cognition or consciousness) was to be prolonged *come what may.* Until the Schiavo case, vitalism was a remnant of ancient or animist faiths. Ultimately, the Schiavo case came to serve as a vehicle for resurgent proselytizing on issues ranging from embryonic stem cell research to abortion.

Ms. Schiavo was in a permanent vegetative state (PVS).[1] That diagnosis was never in doubt among credible medical sources. People in a PVS cannot see, hear, feel. They cannot think.[2] They do not experience or interact purposefully with their environment. In Ms. Schiavo's case, brain scans showed a cerebral cortex filled with spinal fluid. Highly edited videos of her moving and appearing to follow a balloon with her eyes were, to neurologists, clearly bogus. Indeed, neurologists generally looked on with either slack-jawed wonder or incandescent fury at the attempt to deceive the courts and to manipulate the court of public opinion with videos made by those who wanted to prolong her life support. (See the late Ron Cranford's contribution to this volume.) That the videos were indeed deceptive was made bold face when Ms. Schiavo's autopsy results incontrovertibly documented that she suffered from what is called "cortical blindness"—the part of the brain that controls vision had been destroyed. She could not track the movement of a balloon, or anything else, because she could not see the balloon, or anything else. The role and effect of those video images is discussed by several authors in this volume.

Ms. Schiavo was being kept alive by a percutaneous endoscopic gastrostomy (PEG) tube, which delivered a nutrient solution directly to her stomach. During the court battles the tube was removed three times, and reinserted twice.

The dispute between husband Michael Schiavo and parents Robert and Mary Schindler was an awful demonstration of what can go wrong when stakes are high and disputes are hot. The Schindlers, by most accounts sincere and caring, became allied with a variety of partisans who saw in the case a chance to make political hay over everything from "judicial activism" to abortion to creationism to same-sex marriage to stem cell research to end-of-life care itself; some of the "Save Terri" shib-boleths and agit-prop went so far as to suggest that hospice care was active euthanasia in disguise. That, too, is false, but America's Culture Wars too often are about seeking power rather than insight.

Perversely, the case started to unravel a longstanding trans-political and interfaith accord, especially in Florida: Conservatives and liberals had once agreed that there was something wrong when tubes could be stuck—or kept—in people without their consent or that of their next of kin.[3] Moreover, a huge investment in bipartisan, interfaith under-standing was being squandered. The Robert Wood Johnson Foundation had just recently concluded a program to support end-of-life education. Some $150 million had been spent over the previous 15 years, in part with the intention of educating policymakers and legislators. The work of dozens of "Community–State Partnerships" (including one in Florida that included support for the program I direct) was unraveling.

The judge at the center of the case, Pinellas-Pasco County Circuit Court Judge George Greer, consistently ruled in favor of Michael Schiavo, who argued that withdrawal of the PEG tube was what Ms. Schiavo would have wanted. The Schindlers disagreed. Greer endured death threats, relied on bodyguards, and was eventually asked to leave his church.

Michael Schiavo, who later established a political action committee, was similarly reviled by partisans, many of whom alleged, without evidence, that he (a) abused Ms. Schiavo and caused her 1990 collapse, (b) worsened her condition by intentionally waiting to summon help after that collapse, and/or (c) abused her after she was in a PVS. Indeed, in 2005, two-and-a-half months after her death, Florida Governor Jeb Bush asked a state prosecutor to investigate the circumstances of the 1990 cardiac arrest, especially the amount of time that elapsed between Ms. Schiavo's collapse and Mr. Schiavo calling 911. The prosecutors found no evidence of wrongdoing.

None of that dissuaded Mark Fuhrman, the former Los Angeles police detective famous for being the first to arrive at the O.J. Simpson crime scene and finding the bloody glove. Fuhrman, who once admitted to torturing gang members, was seen in a video shown to the Simpson jury in which he repeatedly uttered a racial slur. He later apologized and denied being a racist. His was the first book on the Schiavo case.[4] The book begins, according to the *St. Petersburg Times*, "with a short introduction, explaining that he watched the Schiavo saga from afar and decided to write the book several days after her death. He said he received a telephone call from Sean Hannity, the conservative Fox News talk show host, who asked him to look into the case. Hannity had grown close to Schiavo's parents, Bob and Mary Schindler, while covering the story in Florida. . . . Fuhrman said he wanted to answer several key questions: How did Schiavo collapse? Had she been abused or murdered?"[5]

Since then, several books have been published about the case, almost all of them similarly partisan.[6] The debate across all media was too often about spectacle, too little about illumination.

In a thoroughgoingly sad case, perhaps the saddest aspect was the invocation of disability rights. Those on the political right, traditionally loath to endorse, or at least pay for, reasonable accommodations for people with disabilities, somehow reckoned that Ms. Schiavo was disabled. This produced one of the more paradoxical alliances in American politics: disability rights activists—at the vanguard of one of the most important civil rights movement in a generation—arm-in-arm with far-right-wing politicians, who in some jurisdictions will not build a wheelchair ramp without a court order.[7]

Make no mistake: there was a credible conservative stance on the Schiavo case (and it is expressed superbly by Prof. Daniel Robinson in this volume).[8] The problem was that there was no room for it at the time, given the vehemence and volume of the "Save Terri" machine. The Schiavo case was, for operators of that machine, never about the traditional conservative values of limited government, self-determination, and personal responsibility. It was in part about newly empowered, pre-Obama-era rightists who wanted to revile those they opposed on judicial activism, creationism, and stem cells, issues on which most Americans hold ordinary, that is, not peculiar, views. It was also about a deep and apparently sincere belief that something awful happened when PEG tubes were removed from patients in permanent vegetative states—a belief that no amount of medical evidence could shake.

The Schiavo case will last much longer than Terri Schiavo and, indeed, was an issue through the 2008 U.S. presidential campaign. The politicians who decided there was something in it for them also began to do what legislators are best and worst at: They introduced legislation. In Florida and several other states, laws have been proposed that would invalidate living wills and surrogate refusals of treatment unless such refusals were made explicitly and included the precise future context under which it would be permissible to withdraw or withhold treatment—a burden that as a practical matter would be impossible to meet. PEG tubes are often singled out: The idea is that a surgically implanted tube to deliver a nutrient solution is somehow different than dialysis or ventilator support or antibiotics. Mind you, those advocating "life in any form" tend, at least in Florida, to be unwilling to pay any of the associated costs. As she lay dying, the same Florida Legislature that passed "Terri's Law" to keep her PEG tube from being removed cut the Medicaid budget that pays for the nutrient solution used with PEG tubes to keep patients alive.

While many see Ms. Schiavo's legacy as a greater awareness of living wills, that will be too optimistic if the nation's legislatures succeed in invalidating advance directives and thereby undermine several decades of ecumenical agreement on death and dying. If that happens, it will not be because free people have finally declared solidarity with the vulnerable, affirmed their commitment to life, or taken a stand against over-hasty withholding or withdrawal of life-sustaining treatment. It will be because a narrow band of political outliers framed the debate in such a way as to frighten ordinary people and make them uncertain about what they rightly and sincerely valued.

∷ Right-to-Life and Right-to-Die

This section addresses several core issues in more detail—namely, why the case took its extraordinary course, the controversy over disability, and the role of language in framing debates.

There is something striking about the frequency with which the State of Florida has acquired a significant role in Big Stories (or at least Big Cases). Think Cuban exiles, the missile crisis, and the brink of war (and perhaps the assassination of John F. Kennedy); Watergate and its burglars; the explosion of the Space Shuttle Challenger; Elian; the 2000 presidential election. If state flags were fashioned from grim whimsy, Florida's would be revised to resemble a hanging chad, with a picture of Elian Gonzalez on one side and Terri Schiavo on the other, flapping in a hurricane's gales.

It is not clear whether there really is something about *Florida* that engenders such. Perhaps it is the state's status as a cultural frontier in an era when all geographic frontiers have been used up. Or in the case of protracted legal proceedings it might be coincidence, the tip of a national iceberg shaped by litigation such that there is always one more lawsuit, one more court, one more expert, one more zealot with a filing fee. Then, every once in a while, a case gets so wedged in the courts that it cannot be pried loose. It could happen anywhere.

Some 6,500 people die every day in the United States,[9] and precious few warrant more than a paid death announcement or an agate couplet in the daily paper. End-of-life disputes are common enough, but most of them are resolved by rapprochement, truce, or death. Those cases in which combatants at the death-bedside enjoy no accord, and in which death is reluctant, usually find it is some machine that makes it so. The machines—customarily ventilators, dialysis units, PEG tubes—supplant a vital function and become sine qua nons for life itself. They are good machines, generally speaking.

Indeed, why would one ever disdain such a device?

The "right-to-die" movement, along with hospice, are creatures of the realization that such medical machines are not always tools with which brave people combat death, infrequently ways to help stick one's thumb in the Grim Reaper's eye, rarely means by which one doesn't go gentle into . . . that is, while medical machines can prolong life in extraordinary ways, the lives they prolong are too often dark and bleak and silent, and not particularly valued by anyone without a political train to catch. If one would be dead but for the machine, the machine is a kind of blessing—unless one is not aware enough to know or realize it, and never will. Some clergy have been teaching us this for years, insisting that there is no duty to prolong a life "when the body has become prison to the soul."

Throughout the Schiavo case, those who sought to maintain her on the PEG tube tacitly conceded as much. They did so by denying the accuracy of the PVS diagnosis, and insisting that Ms. Schiavo interacted purposefully with the environment, communicated with loved ones and, generally, had a mental life not significantly different than that of others.[10] This was false, but it was argued with such vehemence that it was clearly a recognition of the fact that if the diagnosis were accurate, then there was little point in postponing the inevitable. That is, if Ms. Schiavo were really in a PVS, then the right thing to do would align with the wishes and desires of any ordinary, reasonable person—and she would be allowed to die.

It would in some respects have been far more interesting if the Schiavo case were a public debate over the deep and interesting questions:

- What is the moral value of the life of a human body that has no human consciousness?
- What are our duties to such a life?
- Can a person while competent make a plausible demand to be maintained indefinitely in a PVS should one occur in the future?
- Beside her PVS, Ms. Schiavo was diagnosed with no malady that would have caused her death. Does *that* make the withdrawal of hydration and nutrition treatment a kind of suicide?

To be sure, those who sought to keep Ms. Schiavo alive were keen to prevail in the courts, and so thoughtful and reasoned end-of-life debate was not a goal. When the diagnosis was bleak, they condemned the physicians. When the family fractured, they assailed the husband. When the rulings went against them, they decried the judges.

∷ Personhood and Process

Many wondered why anti-abortion activists—and the Schiavo case attracted the most extreme and zealous exemplars—would care so much about a non-fetus. What on earth did Terri Schiavo have to do with abortion? The answer can take several paths, but the one with the greatest traction is that, like a fetus, a person in a PVS has no awareness, no cognition, no intentions. As Robin N. Fiore observes in her contribution to this volume, "Theresa Schiavo is recast as a fully accessible fetus: she exhibits arousal without awareness, movement without intention . . ." To be sure, a fetus is in many respects better off than Ms. Schiavo because after a point it does experience sensation. Ms. Schiavo experienced nothing. Further, absent forces to the contrary, a fetus will in the normal course of things become a person; Ms. Schiavo had no such hope. Still, the explanation might go, if Ms. Schiavo and others like her can be taken off life support, then a block has been pulled from the wheels of an engine that will then roll over all life, willy-nilly.

The necessary and sufficient conditions for *personhood* have been a source of great and illuminating debate since antiquity, and that which distinguishes a person from a non-person is and has been a central theme in philosophy. From Boethius (a person is "an individual substance of a rational nature") through Plato, Aristotle and Aquinas, and, in the modern era, from Descartes to Locke to Kant (who likewise emphasized rationality), the analyses of "person" and "personhood" have orbited around reason, rationality, and cognition.[11]

Here, philosophers and ordinary folk reach the same or similar conclusions.[12] If to be a person is to be able to communicate, remember, plan, interact, and reason, and if this is what makes life precious and special, then the permanent absence of an ability to communicate, remember, plan, interact, and reason means that whatever is left has fewer entitlements and protections than those who enjoy full personhood.

This is emphatically not to say that the permanently unconscious have no entitlements and should not be protected. They should be treated in a dignified manner. They should not be abused. They should be accorded some measure of respect. But none of these entitlements includes or entails perpetual medical maintenance. Indeed, if reasonable people generally do not value permanent unconsciousness, one could make the case that perpetual medical maintenance is a moral disservice, the imposition of a device or gadget of the sort dreaded by all those ordinary people who are not ideologues, who don't know much about bioethics and its arguments but who are nonetheless quite clear that they do not want to live or die "on tubes." They believe that such tubes are in fact an affront to dignity, a form of abuse, a diminution of respect. It becomes creepy and perverse to argue that in the absence of an explicit refusal of such indignity, the silence somehow begs for medical intervention. Worse, to suggest that failure to provide the intervention is a form or discrimination or—listen to this—*murder* is to stand in opposition to ordinary moral intuitions, interfaith accord, and social, political, and legal agreement. Alas, that is the unhappy position taken by the zealots who started the Culture Wars. It seemed to be about power and social control, not values or ethics.

The third question asked above—Can a person while competent make a plausible demand to be maintained indefinitely in a PVS should one occur in the future?—is a source of some anxiety. This is because we attach such importance to high-stakes expressions of anticipated future desires. A last will and testament allows me to influence the behavior of others after I am dead; indeed, the law in most cases *requires* the terms of a will be met. If I ask you to bury me on a hill, drink my favorite brandy, or give my fortune to my daughter, then you must do so, *ceteris paribus.* Living wills and other advance directives are additional means to have an influence or to command compliance after the point at which the signer or utterer has lost the ability to interact purposefully with the world. So it has come to be uncontroversial in many contexts to assert that living wills are just as good for requesting future treatment as for denying it. This is a mistake.

One of the most important and paradoxically overlooked distinctions in contemporary bioethics is that between refusals and requests. There is overwhelming and correct agreement that a competent, informed adult who is acting voluntarily can refuse any treatment, service, or intervention she wishes: From breakfast to brain surgery, "no" means "no," even for life-prolonging treatment. This is essential if the concept of informed or valid consent is to be anything but a hollow risk-management stratagem. Morality[13] requires we ask for consent in medicine because we rightly reckon that free agents can and ought to control access to their bodies. But the concept is eviscerated if a competent, free adult cannot also refuse treatment.[14] So, valid refusals are primary and fundamental protections against unwanted medical and other touching.

Requests on the other hand need to be reasonable. One cannot request anything and expect that doing so compels compliance in the same way as a valid refusal. A patient cannot request to be a human subject in a clinical trial, cannot request a dose of morphine for recreational purposes or an antibiotic for a viral infection, cannot request a brain transplant—and expect that the request places any kind of duty on a physician or nurse. So, what kind of reasons might be available to support a request for perpetual medical maintenance in the event of a PVS? There are at least three.

One might suggest that permanent unconsciousness is itself of value. This, as above, is difficult to understand, or believe. What we value about life is consciousness, communication, *interaction*—not simply that we are not dead. One might insist (by slogan rather than argument) that "all human life has value" or "is precious." In such a case, there is really nothing to respond, exactly because it is a slogan. All extraterrestrial life and sea life and bunny life has value, too, depending on how and how precisely we are prepared to define "value." Indeed, we could even accept the sentiment of the slogan but suggest its meager force is worthy of consideration only in cases in which the process of terminating treatment is hasty—obviously not an issue in the Schiavo case. Moreover, such a request attempts to impose extraordinary duties on others. Modern medicine brings us to the point where we can in fact prolong the existence of permanently unconscious humans for quite some time. If requests to do so were in fact reasonable, we should then have to contemplate—and prepare to support financially—the indefinite maintenance of potentially hundreds of thousands of people. This does not look or feel like "respect for the value of life." This looks and feels more like a deliberate attempt to mock it, or to attempt a demonstration of the superiority of our machines over nature's (or God's) processes.

Second, a request for perennial PVS maintenance might also invoke the possibility of future discoveries. That is, a person might express while competent or via a living will a desire to remain on life support (for a while? as long as possible? indefinitely? forever?) in case of a future diagnosis of a PVS because there might be a future treatment that could reverse the diagnosis. Such fantasies are common enough in medicine, and they are usually expressed by the medically desperate or by those prepared to spend hundreds of thousands of dollars to have their heads frozen (large deposit required) by cryonics companies with the expectation they will later be "revivified" and (thereby?) achieve immortality. In fact, though, medical science does not progress in any sort of way that should provide succor. It is slow and accretive. Those both enthralled and encouraged by "gee whiz" news media accounts might thus be deluded into thinking that some breakthrough or other is around the corner for *any* malady. As an argument, therefore, the hope for a future discovery proves too much. It entails—against all evidence—that one ought always to take seriously that if there were just another day of life, then everything would change. As arguments go, it is more to be pitied than scorned.[15]

Another possible reason to request perpetual maintenance is that it might bring comfort or pleasure or even joy to family and friends. Indeed, at a number of points during the case, right-to-life partisans suggested that Mr. Schiavo should relinquish his guardianship authority and duties to the Schindlers, who clearly were prepared to do whatever was necessary to keep Ms. Schiavo alive. The problem with this kind of argument is that it suggests that it is morally permissible to do extraordinary things without consent to a patient for the sake of other people. But we do not permit, for instance, even the harvesting of organs from cadavers for the sake of others without permission in advance from the source of the organs. The idea that it might be acceptable to insert or maintain a tube in someone for the emotional comfort of others, no matter how deep their love, is a bold-face violation of the moral rule that one should not *use* other people. This is Ethics 101, and it is attributed to Immanuel Kant, who held, rightly, that one ought always to treat others as ends in themselves and never as means to an end.[16] This view is quite close to that espoused by many social and political conservatives who want to reject Utilitarian requirements to do the greatest good for the greatest number.[17]

The last of the four questions we are considering here—Does the withdrawal of artificial hydration and nutrition in the absence of any other malady constitute a kind of suicide?—is one that arises even in non-PVS cases. The standard view on this issue is that withholding or withdrawing life-sustaining treatment constitutes a getting-out-of-the-way of the dying process. A patient with end-stage kidney disease who forgoes dialysis dies because of the kidney disease; a heart attack patient who refuses cardiopulmonary resuscitation dies because of heart disease; a pneumonia patient who insists that ventilator support be removed dies of pneumonia. But withdrawing Ms. Schiavo's PEG tube allowed no independent fatal process to overwhelm her. The argument may be put this way:[18]

1. If a patient has no underlying malady that would lead to death, and
2. Withdrawing or withholding medical hydration and nutrition will lead to death, then
3. Withholding or withdrawal in such cases must involve the *intent* to cause death (perhaps a good death); therefore,
4. A capacitated person's successful intent to bring about one's own death is suicide, and a surrogate's successful intent to bring about another person's death is assisted suicide.

But this illicitly overlooks other reasonable and plausible intentions. For instance, PEG tube refusal in the absence of a distinct fatal malady might be motivated by any of a number of rational desires or intentions. That is, by refusing a PEG tube, one might one might intend primarily to:

1. Refuse an invasive procedure, or
2. Avoid running any of the risks of tube placement or maintenance, or
3. Make a political point, or
4. Exercise personal liberty, or
5. Express and act upon an unwillingness to forgo *eating*, or
6. Express and act upon the view that PEG tubes reduce dignity . . . and so on.

Now, none of these intentions involves intending to die (or bring about death), even though it is known that dying will follow from any of them being acted on. This is not intending to die, any more than a parent, say, *intends* to die by interposing himself between a child and a deadly force; or a soldier *intends* to die by doing something brave and foreseeably fatal. The intention of these acts is not to *cause* one's own or another's death, even as the act is a sufficient condition for the death.

It might be objected that some of the reasons here exaggerate the burdens of PEG insertion and maintenance and under-emphasize the concomitant burdens on family members and society.[19] But the point here is that this larger debate was not engaged, perhaps partly out of shyness by those who knew morality either permitted or required removal of Ms. Schiavo's PEG tube and were reluctant to argue that even the intent to cause one's or another's death *in such circumstances* is itself not blameworthy. To do so would have been to risk allowing "save Terri" advocates to exult—with the cameras rolling—that the case was really about assisted suicide after all. They would have been mistaken, but that would not be discovered in public in the absence of reasoned debate, or in the presence of political and religious advocacy.

What should be clear is that the overarching *ethical* issues raised by the Schiavo case had been resolved well before the case made the evening news, especially that:

- People and their surrogates have the right to refuse medical treatment.
- What we value about life is not merely the absence of death.
- Irrational desires do not impose bona fide duties on health professionals.

So how, in the face of broad agreement, did the Schiavo disagreement come to take its extraordinary and ugly course?

:: Money, Politics, and Zealotry

By most accounts, Bob and Mary Schindler, Ms. Schiavo's parents, were dedicated and compassionate. It is an awful thing to lose a child, and they fought vigorously. Michael Schiavo and the Schindlers got along well from 1990, when Ms. Schiavo collapsed during heart failure, apparently as a result of an eating disorder, to 1993, when a malpractice jury awarded $300,000 to Mr. Schiavo and about $700,000 to Ms. Schiavo. The relationship deteriorated, and in 1993 the Schindlers attempted to have Mr. Schiavo removed as guardian. From 1994 to 1998, they disagreed over the level of Ms. Schiavo's care. In 1998, Mr. Schiavo petitioned the court to authorize the removal of Ms. Schiavo's PEG tube; the Schindlers opposed him, saying that she would want to remain alive. The trial began in January 2000, with Pinellas-Pasco County Circuit Court Judge Greer presiding.

During the trial, the Schindlers were adamant—passionate—in expressing the view that there were no circumstances under which they would ever agree to withdrawing the PEG tube or, indeed, any other form of treatment. University of South Florida professor Jay Wolfson, appointed as guardian *ad litem* in October 2003, observed this in his report to Governor Bush:

> Testimony provided by members of the Schindler family included very personal statements about their desire and intention to ensure that Theresa remain alive. Throughout the course of the litigation, deposition and trial testimony by members of the Schindler family voiced the disturbing belief that they would keep Theresa alive at any and all costs. Nearly gruesome examples were given, eliciting agreement by family members that in the event Theresa should contract diabetes and subsequent gangrene in each of her limbs, they would agree to amputate each limb, and would then, were she to be diagnosed with heart disease, perform open heart surgery. There was additional, difficult testimony that appeared to establish that despite the sad and undesirable condition of Theresa, the parents still derived joy from having her alive, even if Theresa might not be at all aware of her environment given the persistent vegetative state. Within the testimony, as part of the hypotheticals presented, Schindler family members stated that even if Theresa had told them of her intention to have artificial nutrition withdrawn, they would not do it. Throughout this painful and difficult trial, the family acknowledged that Theresa was in a diagnosed persistent vegetative state.[20]

Such impassioned parental advocacy was neither new nor a surprise. Family members of loved ones in permanent vegetative states often both believe they are somehow communicating with them and reckon that anything less than never-say-die advocacy constitutes failure or abandonment, or both. The Schindlers' perseverance in the courts was noted by various news media, which were in turn noticed by what Jon Eisenberg calls "the right-wing think-tank machinery":

> I heeded the advice given by Mark "Deep Throat" Felt to *Washington Post* reporters Bob Woodward and Carl Bernstein during the Watergate scandal: "Follow the money." I began to study the right-wing think-tank machinery and trace its funding of advocates for Bob and Mary Schindler and Governor Jeb Bush. I was increasingly amazed as I learned that nearly everyone on the Schindler-Bush team was somehow connected—mostly

financially, sometimes in other ways—with one or more right-wing foundations and think tanks. [My assistant] was right. It was, as she put it, "one big web of donations and grants"—and the *Schiavo* case was smack in the middle of the web.[21]

The Schiavo case would not—could not—have taken its extraordinary and lengthy course if it had not been adopted and paid for by partisans whose day jobs involved promoting prayer in schools, creationism, and tax cuts, and opposing stem cell research, "activist judges," and gay adoptions. Terri Schiavo had become a cause. There was a kind of precedent for this, too. Ms. Schiavo's heart failed on Feb. 25, 1990. On that day, and since 1983, Nancy Cruzan was in a PVS in Missouri, where right-to-life Governor John Ashcroft, later President George W. Bush's attorney general, fought to keep her alive, much like President Bush's brother, Governor Jeb Bush, did for Ms. Schiavo. Ms. Cruzan's PEG tube was removed when the legal process ran its course, and she died on Christmas Day, 1990. But it wasn't merely Governor Ashcroft's conservative zeal that provides a parallel. It was the onslaught of spurious and desperate litigation that gave Schiavo viewers such a strong sense of déjà vu: Religious rightists haranguing judges, anti-abortion extremists on the picket lines and ululating sound bites suggesting that withdrawing medical treatment somehow equaled killing.

Listen to William Colby, the Cruzan-family lawyer, describe the events four days before Ms. Cruzan's death:

> The judge told me that someone would let me know about the hearing. Thirty minutes later, his law clerk called to say that the judge had canceled it. Soon after, they faxed over his one-page ruling, which dismissed the case and cautioned the protesters that any further filings could be an abuse of process. *Good for the judge,* I thought as I read his order . . . In front of the courthouse, Randall Terry talked to a small group of reporters, but canceling the hearing had in fact deflated Operation Rescue's publicity balloon. [Judge] "Whipple is a coward," Terry shouted, "and I hope history remembers him as such. Isn't there a judge in this whole blessed state who has the integrity to stand up for this woman?" . . . The Missouri Supreme Court quickly dismissed the new filing as well, and [state trial court] Judge [Byron] Kinder listened only briefly to a protestor's plea before interrupting. "I just despise people like you," he said. "Get out of here." The judiciary had apparently had enough of these protestors.[22]

A decade and a half later, Mr. Terry was hired by the Terri Schindler Schiavo Foundation, set up by her parents and siblings, to organize protests and otherwise advance the cause. "I promise you, if she dies, there will be hell to pay," he said after Ms. Schiavo's PEG tube was removed, and before he mounted a primary election challenge against Jim King, a Republican in the Florida Senate who voted against state intervention in the case.[23] Mr. Terry also had turned on Governor Bush, who, when all the appeals ran out, finally gave up. Bush later endorsed King, who won handily in 2006.

Mr. Terry's defeat in Florida was but one sign that ordinary people were not prepared to purchase the "Save Terri" line of religious right/neocon life-enhancement products. At the national level, however, the lesson took longer to learn. In March and April 2005, during the most awful heat of the Schiavo frenzy, it seemed to some that this permanently unconscious woman could be used to make political hay. Here is the text of a memo circulated by Republican senators on the political advantages of supporting legislation to reinsert Ms. Schiavo's nutrition tube. (The text is quoted verbatim and without corrections: the actual bill number is S. 539 and Ms. Schiavo's first name is misspelled in the first line):

S. 529, The Incapacitated Person's Legal Protection Act

- Teri Schiavo is subject to an order that her feeding tubes will be disconnected on March 18, 2005 at 1 p.m.
- The Senate needs to act this week, before the Budget Act is pending business, or Terri's family will not have a remedy in federal court.
- This is an important moral issue and the pro-life base will be excited that the Senate is debating this important issue.
- This is a great political issue, because Senator Nelson of Florida has already refused to become a cosponsor and this is a tough issue for Democrats.
- The bill is very limited and defines custody as "those parties authorized or directed by a court order to withdraw or withhold food, fluids, or medical treatment."
- There is an exemption for a proceeding "which no party disputes, and the court finds, that the incapacitated person while having capacity, had executed a written advance directive valid under applicably law that clearly authorized the withholding or withdrawal of food or fluids or medical treatment in the applicable circumstances."
- Incapacitated persons are defined as those "presently incapable of making relevant decisions concerning the provision, withholding or withdrawal of food fluids or medical treatment under applicable state law."
- This legislation ensures that individuals like Terri Schiavo are guaranteed the same legal protections as convicted murderers like Ted Bundy.[24]

One does not need to await a future historical assessment to see that while Ms. Schiavo's misfortune was cast as a matter of right-to-life principle, it is most accurately seen as an opportunity to advance a political agenda. When it backfired, there was no choice but to recant.

U.S. Senator Mel Martinez (R-Florida) later admitted that the whole approach was wrong—or at least politically ineffective—and that federal courts should not intervene in such intimate matters; he nevertheless opined that it was permissible for state courts to intervene.[25] Given the issues at stake, such an opinion makes a distinction without a difference: How much does it matter which government intervenes in bedside disputes?

The duel, and its echo of the Cruzan case, continued to the graveside. When Nancy Cruzan was buried in 1990, her grave marker was adapted from an editorial cartoon by Steve Benson that included the jagged lines of a medical monitor display spelling out the words "thank you" and then flattening out.[26] Then:

> Born: July 20, 1957
> Departed: January 11, 1983
> At Peace: December 26, 1990

Mr. Benson repeated the theme a decade and a half later, with an editorial cartoon showing a monitor next to Ms. Schiavo's bedside, the display reading "thank you Michael" before flattening out. Ms. Schiavo's gravestone in Clearwater, Florida, reads in part:

> Born December 3, 1963
> Departed This Earth
> February 25, 1990
> At Peace March 31, 2005

∷ Schiavo and Disability

On March 18, 2005, the U.S. House of Representatives Committee on Government Reform issued five subpoenas: one commanding Michael Schiavo to appear before it and bring with him the "hydration and nutrition equipment" in working order; three calling for physicians and other personnel at Ms. Schiavo's hospice to do the same; and one commanding Ms. Schiavo to appear. The subpoenas would require that the PEG tube remain in working order until at least the date of testimony, March 25, 2005. The idea—the very idea—that a person who had been in a PVS for 15 years could be subpoenaed to testify before the U.S. House of Representatives was as breathtakingly strange as anything that had occurred in the case.[27]

Next to being asked to testify, one of the strangest and most troubling aspects of the Schiavo case was its adoption as a cause célèbre by the militant wing of the disability rights community, elements of which regarded Ms. Schiavo as a member of that community. This was troublesome for several reasons:

1. It was based on no coherent definition of disability.
2. It appeared to be politically motivated—with the paradoxical effect of a group deserving special accommodations allying with partisans who previously showed no special interest in disability rights or helping people with disabilities.
3. It had the effect of reducing the rights of people with disabilities to refuse burdensome treatment.

We should consider these in turn.

Was Terri Schiavo Disabled?

The long and unhappy history of the devaluation of handicapped people or people with disabilities has produced a movement that seeks improved social and medical services; public accommodations for things like wheelchair access, Braille translations, and personal assistance; and antidiscrimination laws and policies. Most of these are in large part uncontroversial. They are based on the idea that people with disabilities *need* such help and that civilized society ought to provide it. (Lawrence Nelson's contribution to this volume provides an excellent and comprehensive analysis.)

Progress in achieving such social changes has been made despite no clear agreement on what kind of conceptual model is most appropriate for defining disability in the first place. Most generally, two models are invoked: the medical model, which holds that people with disabilities are in some way physiologically harmed such that they are unable in varying degrees to do or experience things that other people do or experience, and the social model, which emphasizes society's response to and attribution of capacity to people with different capacities.[28]

It can be especially difficult to come to agreement on a definition of cognitive disability. The American Association on Mental Retardation, for instance, holds that:

> Mental retardation is not something you have, like blue eyes, or a bad heart. Nor is it something you are, like short, or thin. It is not a medical disorder, nor a mental disorder. Mental retardation is a particular state of functioning that begins in childhood and is characterized by limitation in both intelligence and adaptive skills. Mental retardation reflects the "fit" between the capabilities of individuals and the structure and expectations of their environment.[29]

There is no sense, of course, in which Terri Schiavo had mental retardation. But the notion of a "limitation in both intelligence and adaptive skills" seems to capture the core idea of a cognitive or mental impairment such that one thus affected may be said to be "disabled." Put differently, *any* kind of disability must involve a limitation, an impairment, a decreased function of some sort. To be sure, there are groups that deny that impaired or lost function constitutes disability at all,[30] but this provides no comfort for the partisans who were keen to keep Ms. Schiavo alive—they *needed* her to be disabled in order to enlist the political and economic support of disability rights groups.

There is no coherent definition of "disability" that can apply to Ms. Schiavo or anyone else in a PVS. To be permanently unconscious is not to have *limitations, impediments,* or *decreased functions.* It is to have nothing: The awful fact is that Ms. Schiavo, according to the series of neurologists who examined her, had no non-autonomic functions at all. There was no experience, activity, or sensation such that with assistance or reasonable accommodation or special support she would have been able to have, do, or feel; and, with one exception, there is no biological (let alone human) function that can be provided for her. The exception is hydration and nutrition, without which she died. To regard Ms. Schiavo as disabled was a perverse disservice to the millions of people who need assistance with tasks involving moving, hearing, seeing, even thinking. With assistance, they can accomplish and experience many things. By diagnostic definition, Ms. Schiavo could accomplish nothing, experience nothing, do nothing. Moreover and alas, she never would have been able to. This would be an insult if directed at someone with a bona fide disability. In Ms. Schiavo's case it was a description of a tragedy.

Even the term "disabled" is often condemned as implying that handicapped people have *no* abilities, and for this reason some people prefer the descriptor "differentially abled." Derided in some quarters for its air of political correctness, the term in fact makes an important distinction between those with limitations and those with no abilities whatsoever. If Terri Schiavo were to be regarded as disabled, she was utterly different than the millions of constituents of the differentially abled rights groups that have so successfully—and correctly—changed society and changed its laws.

Unusual Politics
All of which makes it mysterious that such groups had been beguiled into thinking that Terri Schiavo could be a member, and that allowing her to die was somehow an affront to people with disabilities.

For years, a variety of ultra-conservative, anti-abortion, and anti-right-to-die groups fought to prevent the withdrawal of Ms. Schiavo's PEG tube. Some of these organizations link abortion with both assisted suicide and what had only recently been uncontroversial—the voluntary withdrawal or withholding of medical treatment. Some even suggested that hospice care is somehow like active euthanasia or assisted suicide.[31] As above, it is not clear why the anti-abortion movement would care about Terri Schiavo, or why there would even be an anti-hospice movement. One explanation is just that these partisans are socially conservative and they believe, falsely, that the hospice and right-to-die movements are liberal. Another is that they are vitalists, or believers in the transcendent value of non-sentient human life. If life must be protected and prolonged come what may, then not only must the life of the fetus be protected, but hospice must be stopped because some people there die sooner than they would have otherwise.

For whatever reason, these groups decided that Ms. Schiavo was someone who should not be allowed to die. What is most striking, though, is that they somehow convinced many in the disability community of this. This sad alliance evolved in spite of the fact that the conservatives in the right-to-life and anti-assisted-suicide movements and their legislative allies have never been strong supporters of disability rights. Indeed, people with disabilities are regarded by at least some conservatives as constituting just another interest group seeking special treatment—and tax support—from legislatures. In Florida, a legislature that consistently has been less than responsive to the needs of people with developmental disabilities, among others, somehow accepted the notion that Terri Schiavo was disabled and in 2003 passed "Terri's Law" authorizing the governor to stay a court order requiring the re-insertion of Ms. Schiavo's PEG tube.[32] This was taken to be a great victory by some in the disability community—a community that should probably not expect such an outpouring of legislative concern and support to include increased tax funding to help provide services otherwise unavailable to its constituents. Moreover, subsequent legal efforts by the governor and others explicitly made the case that court rulings that would lead to removal of Ms. Schiavo's PEG tube constitute discrimination against handicapped people.

The anti-abortion link to the disability rights movement is clearer than to PVS and Ms. Schiavo. Some in the disability movement have come out strongly against (some) abortions because it can be seen as a way to kill fetuses that would become persons with disabilities.

It follows that many sorts of genetic tests on fetuses are likewise to be disdained. All this is despite the fact that many ardent supporters of what has been called the "disability rights critique" otherwise support abortion rights.[33] Relatedly, the disability community has an interest in opposing active euthanasia and assisted suicide by virtue of the history of Nazis and others killing people with disabilities—*lebensunwerten Lebens*—or those "lives unworthy of life." Among the ugliest scenes in the Schiavo drama, some of those involved in the legal conflict over Ms. Schiavo were compared to anti-disability Nazis.

It is difficult to disentangle these alliances. What emerges, however, is that some elements of a disability community that has rarely enjoyed the help or support of social conservatives had been convinced by those conservatives that they had an interest in the outcome of Ms. Schiavo's case; or perhaps that they could use the conservative movement in the service of disability rights; or both. A consortium of disability groups in 2003 declared that:

> The "right to life" movement has embraced her as a cause to prove "sanctity of life." The "right-to-die" movement believes she is too disabled to live and therefore better off dead. Yet the life-and-death issues surrounding Terri Schindler-Schiavo are first and foremost disability rights issues—issues which affect millions of Americans with disabilities, old and young. . . . Can she think? Hear? Communicate? These questions apply to thousands of people with disabilities who, like Ms. Schindler-Schiavo, cannot currently articulate their views and so must rely on others as substitute decision-makers . . . [34]

Of course, supporters of Michael Schiavo did not suggest that Ms. Schiavo *or anyone else* is "too disabled to live." Merely to suggest that they did is to succumb to extremist agit-prop. But the slogans and invective fail unless Ms. Schiavo can be made out to be "disabled person" rather than a dying person.

May Disabled People Refuse Treatment?

It is therefore sad and mysterious that disability activists chose thus to ally with the religious right that previously had shown little interest in their causes, rather than with the more moderate disabled groups that work for parity with respect to medical decision making, including choices in dying. Saddest of all, perhaps, is that by partnering with political extremists, the actions of the disability community—not unlike the Florida Legislature—bid fair to set back a quarter-century of progress in strengthening the right of people to refuse treatment.

Most everyone rightly agrees that informed, capacitated, uncoerced adults can refuse any treatment they like, including life-sustaining treatment. The foundations of informed or valid consent are feckless and useless unless valid refusal enjoys equal status. Matters are complicated when individuals lose capacity, but even this has been addressed by the evolution of surrogacy and proxy decision making. However imperfect in certain circumstances, the role of surrogates solves many problems related to consent and refusal. Now, the "save Terri" partisans were not in all cases opposed to valid refusal of treatment. What they seemed to oppose is surrogate refusal, which is why Ms. Schiavo's husband was the target of such heated calumny. The goal in some quarters was to prevail with the idea that absent a living will that explicitly refuses artificial hydration and nutrition, there are no grounds to terminate such treatment.

But this stance constitutes a tacit insistence that of the legal standards for surrogate decision making—substituted judgment, best interests, and reasonable person—only substituted judgment is morally acceptable. The consequences of allowing this notion to prevail would be extraordinary. Indeed, the Florida Legislature in 2004 considered, and fortunately rejected, a measure that would have required advance, explicit, written refusal of artificial hydration and nutrition before these treatments could in fact be withheld or removed. The success of such measures would have meant that a loving surrogate could not use the best-interests standard to request withdrawal of a PEG tube. The thrust of these efforts misses the fact that after a decade and a half of permanent unconsciousness, most reasonable people would in fact choose to terminate the medical intervention prolonging such an existence; and hence that their surrogates should be able to as well.

Should people with disabilities be troubled by this argument? It is not clear why, at least on ethical grounds. If people *without* disabilities have and often exercise the right to refuse treatment, and their surrogates, proxies, or guardians have the right to do so on their behalf, then why shouldn't people *with* disabilities enjoy the same right? If there are no ethical grounds to prevent people with disability from refusing treatment, there might however be historical or political grounds. In some jurisdictions, disability groups insist that surrogates for hospital patients who are disabled must *never* authorize withholding or withdrawal of treatment, for that would constitute premature ending of the life of a person with a disability—à la the Nazis, again. Unfortunately, these groups hew to this policy *even when the patient has a serious malady unrelated to the disability.* In other words, once a person is disabled, she cannot through a representative refuse any medical intervention at all; she cannot use the services of hospice; and so she cannot enjoy what has—paradoxically, since Nuremberg—been the right to say no.

This bit of paternalism would be inoffensive if there were any reason to believe that the people it is supposed to protect would really want the protection. As it is, we are left with the unfounded suggestion *qua* policy that disabled people have fewer or lesser interests in forgoing burdensome treatment than people without disabilities, a suggestion for which there was no argument and, apparently, no evidence.[35]

:: Ethics, Culture, and Language

As the Schiavo case evolved, its extraordinary status was made clear by the lengths to which the executive and legislative branches of the governments of Florida and the United States were prepared to go to prevent the termination of medical care, a termination that occurs thousands of times a day without controversy in the United States and many other countries. It was as if agents of those branches were using litigation and legislation as weapons they thought could and should prove dispositive, firing them in a display of overwhelming force. They might as well have made rubber stamps for legal motions and petitions reading *Ultima ratio regum,* or "the last argument of kings," reminding their Culture Wars opponents of Louis XIV and the motto he affixed to cannon.

But "the state" in democracies is not monolithic, and the idea that force or, what is sometimes indistinguishable, legal bullying, might be appropriate is as wrong-headed as it is tempting. At least as striking as the frequency of spurious legal filings and peculiar legislation was how consistently the judicial branch of government wouldn't have any of it. Indeed, the only times Ms. Schiavo's parents or their allies seemed to prevail in court were in fact examples of judges bending over backwards to avoid being accused of being over-hasty, biased, or incautious.

That the "save Terri" camp could not win a ruling that mattered was seen by some as evidence in support of the notion that judges were not merely interpreting law but making it, from the bench. This is the essence of the complaint over "judicial activism." The scare quotes are needed because it is a phrase designed to communicate the idea that such a thing, whatever it is, is bad.[36] It is bad because it flies in the face of the standard picture of judges as above it all, impartial, and unconcerned by matters not related to critical analysis of precedent. Now, if you oppose certain judicial rulings on *political* grounds, and can make the label "activist" stick, it marks judges you don't like as doing something wrong. So, from abortion to prayer in schools, rulings disdained by social and some other conservatives are taken to warrant claims that activist judges are leading the country astray.

But "judicial activism" was only one of many terms and phrases, some quite ordinary, that were misapplied, misused, and as a result misunderstood by journalists and the lay public. In some cases, the misuse was intentional and designed to deceive. In others, pre-existing semantic ambiguity or vagueness was exploited to similar effect.[37] In many respects, this confusion is evidence of an inability of journalists to accomplish what they tend to say they must accomplish: see through the smoke and give readers or viewers an undistorted view of the world, providing unbiased interpretation when required. There is unfortunately a long history of journalists failing at this, perhaps especially in scientific matters:

> Not only do journalists tend to present science with relatively few caveats, few sources, and little historical context, according to studies, but they also appear more interested in the carefully crafted results (or products) that scientists produce than in the messy, interpretative and often very social processes by which they are produced.[38]

It should therefore be expected that hospice-parking-lot spectacles and who-wins-and-loses court decisions are going to receive greater attention than analysis of the meaning of a cortical encephalogram in a patient with extensive brain damage. Ms. Schiavo's cortical brain scan was flat, meaning, according to neurologists, that she was cortically dead. Were it the case that her brainstem also showed no electrical activity, then, according to nearly universally accepted criteria, she would have been brain dead. In their contribution to this volume, Professors Jay Black and Robert Walker review a number of important issues related to media coverage of the Schiavo case.

A review of some particularly significant words and phrases that were misused or caused misunderstandings in the Schiavo case demonstrates the way language can shape—or warp—debate.

"Brain Death"

The definition of death itself is a source of extensive medical and ethical analysis. The evolution of machines that could supplant respiration and circulation complicated the use of either of those criteria to define death, and the new science of organ transplantation called for definitions and tests that would permit the timely harvesting of organs.[39] What emerged was neurological and not cardiopulmonary: the whole-brain-death criterion. This was first laid out in the Harvard Report, taken up by a presidential commission, and addressed by the National Conference of Commissioners on Uniform State Laws.[40] All states and many countries now adopt some form of whole-brain death, such that with a valid diagnosis of brain death a patient is regarded as, well, dead. At that, some conservative religious organizations refuse to accept the criterion.

The phrase "brain death" was misused during the Schiavo case by those who wanted to suggest that because Ms. Schiavo was not brain dead, any sort of termination of her treatment was inappropriate. This is an instance of a misunderstanding tricked out to appear as an argument. Ms. Schiavo was not brain dead, and no one knowingly suggested she was. By noting this fact in the way some did, the implication was that brain death is required, or is a precondition, for terminating treatment.

That of course is false, but it appeared designed to confuse the ignorant and make it seem like efforts to withdraw the PEG tube were inappropriate and over-hasty. It is also possible that those who tried to take the "But she's not brain dead!" line actually misunderstood the meaning of it themselves. When that was the case, they were not acting deceptively; they were just wrong.

"Err on the Side of Life"

In circumstances shaped by uncertainty and high stakes, what could be more reasonable than caution? What should guide us more than the desire to manage error? When it came to Ms. Schiavo, why not err on the side of life?

That phrase was uttered repeatedly by then-President George W. Bush and others.[41] The problem with such a stance in cases such as Ms. Schiavo's is that it proves too much—much too much. Without further explanation or justification, the claim sounds so reasonable that one must err on the side of life in all cases, whatever it means and come what may. One would *never* be able to terminate any treatment; one would *regularly* have to offer (and pay for) any treatment, no matter how little evidence supported it; one would *always* have to vote (enthusiastically) in favor of any tax increase if there were even a small chance that doing so might reduce mortality for even a single citizen.

Additionally, to err on the side of anything requires that there be uncertainty about the facts and the consequences. Why err on the side of life for Ms. Schiavo given the evidence that her life was bleak, that most people would not value it, that there was evidence adequate to the courts that she herself did not want it, etc.? Why not err on the side of dignity or liberty or privacy? "Err on the side of life" is one of those phrases used in politically fraught circumstances as a kind of moral blunt object: One objects to it on pain of being accused of opposing nothing less than life itself. As an example of framing the Schiavo debate, "side of life" claims were nearly as pervasive as "starvation" allegations.

"Feeding Tube"

"Feeding" is the giving of food. "Food," in ordinary language, is the stuff we *eat* (as opposed to liquids, which we *drink*). Food provides nutrition, sustenance, and so we are happy to permit metaphoric uses that include machines to provide nutrition and therefore sustenance. Hence "feeding tube," or, generally, a tube inserted through the skin and abdominal wall during a percutaneous endoscopic gastrostomy, or nasogastric tubes, which are inserted through the nose. The problem here stems from ordinary associations of feeding with food—meaning that withdrawing a tube that provides nutrition becomes something awful, as if removing it were somehow like snatching a spoon out of your mouth.

That hand was played to good effect during the Schiavo case, where medically administered artificial hydration and nutrition was regularly presented as something ordinary, thus making its withdrawal extraordinary. In fact, the withholding or withdrawal of artificial nutrition and hydration is generally and correctly regarded as not unlike the withholding or withdrawing of any other medical treatment, including other life-sustaining or -prolonging treatment.[42] Moreover, there is evidence in some populations that artificial nutrition and hydration poses serious and sometimes life-threatening risks and so is often contraindicated.[43] In other words, the mere availability of the treatment does not automatically impose on physicians and others a duty to use it.

At end, the picture that was painted showed husband Michael seeking permission from the courts to have Ms. Schiavo's tube removed because he wanted to kill her. When the courts agreed, it became "judicial murder."[44] Fortunately, such hyperbole was so shrill and rang so false, it seemed to have no effect on most ordinary people—people who might have come to fear their final days could be scripted by political and religious activists.

"Starvation"

The case's most extensively misused term was "starvation." Indeed, it is arguable that but for this word the case would not have become the political free-for-all it did. If Mr. Schiavo wanted to kill his wife, the means was "starving her to death." It sounded dreadful.

"Starve" has several senses, two of which matter here. One is simply to perish from lack of nutrition; the other is the affect or feeling of being very, very hungry. Anyone who has missed breakfast and lunch might be forgiven for saying, come mid-afternoon, "I'm starving." It was this sense that was proffered as a reason why the PEG tube should not have been removed. If you feel that awful having missed breakfast and lunch, imagine how that poor Ms. Schiavo will feel after a week or two! The repeated and extensive use of the term was disingenuous precisely because it was designed to elicit sympathy and promote empathy.

In fact, according to neurologists, Ms. Schiavo's brain was so extensively damaged that she was unable to have any sensation of hunger.

In fact, it is well known that many other kinds of patients, as well as people who voluntarily stop eating (as on hunger strikes), actually suffer little because of the natural production of brain ketones, which serve as an anesthetic and can dramatically reduce discomfort from lack of nutrition.[45]

In fact, artificial hydration and nutrition is one of several life-prolonging medical interventions that are halted frequently and without conflict or discomfort.

It follows that suggesting that something terrible is happening when artificial hydration and nutrition are withheld or withdrawn is therefore to embrace the idea that one ought never to do so. But this is preposterous. We regularly stop ventilator support, and no one says a patient is being suffocated; we regularly halt dialysis treatment, and no one says a patient is being poisoned; we regularly cease antibiotic and chemotherapeutic treatments, and no one says a patient is being neglected. This is all because what we value is life, not machines or biochemistry. Peter Schwartz put it best: "What is sacred is life, after all, not medical intervention."[46]

"Vegetative State"

In 1807, J.C. Reil proposed a new term, *vegetative Nervensystem*, because it seemed that the system was chiefly concerned with the organs and functions of nutrition, known since the 17th century as vegetative. "Vegetative nervous system" has survived to the present day.[47]

To be sure, "vegetative state" is a metaphor, but a longstanding one, and no one need take offense. But that is exactly what happened. Ms. Schiavo's diagnosis of PVS came to be taken as an affront, an insult: she was a *vegetable*, and so that made it OK to take away from her what human beings need to live. In March 2004, Pope John Paul II, who himself died shortly after Ms. Schiavo when *he* was taken off life support, addressed the World Federation of Catholic Medical Associations and Pontifical Academy for Life Congress. His remarks were widely reported:

> Faced with patients in similar clinical conditions, there are some who cast doubt on the persistence of the "human quality" itself, almost as if the adjective "vegetative" (whose use is now solidly established), which symbolically describes a clinical state, could or should be instead applied to the sick as such, actually demeaning their value and personal dignity. In this sense, it must be noted that this term, even when confined to the clinical context, is certainly not the most felicitous when applied to human beings. . . . In opposition to such trends of thought, I feel the duty to reaffirm strongly that the intrinsic value and personal dignity of every human being do not change, no matter what the concrete circumstances of his or her life. *A man, even if seriously ill or disabled in the exercise of his highest functions, is and always will be a man,* and he will never become a "vegetable" or an "animal" . . . Even our brothers and sisters who find themselves in the clinical condition of a "vegetative state" retain their human dignity in all its fullness.[48]

He was right, of course: A man is always a man. Human beings are not vegetables. No humans, including those who are very sick, ever (should) lose their dignity. If any of those who advocated for the withdrawal of Ms. Schiavo's PEG tube did so because they undervalued her humanity as a result of a 200-year-old medical term, then they erred. On the other hand, many of those advocates contended that if Ms. Schiavo suffered any indignity, it was because her cognitive darkness and silence prevented her from reaching what most people would seek: deliverance, peace, and some sort of assurance that videos of her in that state would not be made and used to deceive lawmakers and others.

∷ Conclusion

While the Schiavo case served to spark discussion about ethics and end-of-life care, about disability, about the role of government in family disputes, about life and death—it was not itself a dispute driven by reasoned disagreement about values or issues in moral philosophy or contemporary problems in bioethics. It was about power and politics. It was moved forward by political and religious activists, it was litigated by political and religious activists, it was on the front pages because of political and religious activism (when have we ever seen the news media take such an interest in philosophical issues?).

Those who wanted to "save Terri" therefore wanted much more, as well. They wanted to use the power of the government they otherwise disdained to advance a suite of conservative causes. Believers, generally, that the United States is and should be a "Judeo-Christian" (or sometimes just Christian) nation, they wanted to use the case to foster the primacy of certain social, political, and religious values. Ms. Schiavo became an unwilling prop in the Culture Wars, her hospice a place for those who never worried about hunger as a social issue to worry about hers, a vast "moral resort area" (in Saul Bellow's phrase) for those who wanted to get that sweet feel of social engagement and political involvement. Would that the energy spent on Schiavo, the case, have been dedicated to ending poverty or discrimination or real hunger by people who are not unconscious, or to providing social services to those whose actual disabilities could be ameliorated.

While the partisans managed to beguile governors, legislators, and a President, they lost, and endured no small ridicule in the process. This is due to an independent judiciary and so ultimately a tribute to the separation of powers in the United States. But even the courts took a beating, and there is growing evidence that some judges now fear being "Schiavoed," or subjected to intense litigation and threats in disputed end-of-life or other "values" cases.

The best that can be hoped for is not so bad: Millions of ordinary people tried to imagine what it would be like to be unconscious forever, and they talked to their friends and families in a great, international there-but-for-the-grace-of-God-go-I thought experiment. If that continues, and if the world's legislatures do not conflate "commitment to the vulnerable" with intubating the unconscious, or "respect for life" with denying the values of the living, then Ms. Schiavo's legacy provides countless teaching moments and learning opportunities. As legacies go, the rest of us including those of us in the bioethics community who spout off at the deathbeds of strangers, should be so lucky.

∷ Overview of the Rest of the Book

One of the goals of this volume is to provide a broad, critical survey of the issues raised by the Schiavo case. Contributors therefore include those directly involved in the case, as well as those who watched it from afar. Most have clear opinions about its direction and outcome, and several viewpoints are represented. It is hoped that such diversity will inform and guide future debate.

In Chapter 2, Jay Wolfson describes and comments on his experience as Ms. Schiavo's guardian. The opportunity to serve was extraordinary and unparalleled. Prof. Wolfson met all principals in the case and spent extensive time with Ms. Schiavo. Melding his personal experiences with his concerns for social justice, he writes, "The Schiavo case screamed to me about values and convictions, personal and family decisions, the defining of life and death—but it also spoke volumes about how we as individuals and as a nation make heart-wrenching decisions about the allocation of scarce medical resources."

Chapter 3 provides a thoughtful, politically and socially conservative analysis of the issues raised by the case. Daniel Robinson's view—that some basic issues "were either ignored or systematically misunderstood by the cadre of bioethicists, physicians and lawyers willing, if not eager, to inform the nation by way of sound-bites and fleeting interviews"—is a must-read for liberals and others who took an overly facile stance toward the facts and issues in the case.

Kathy Cerminara provides in Chapter 4 a thorough review of the legal course of the case, and then projects the case's effects on future law. In a positive and wise conclusion, she writes, "More education in the law of end-of-life decision-making would help lessen some of these practical effects on judges, legislators and the citizenry. . . . more education would help judges feel prepared to hear cases and to produce considered results even in the face of heated reactions such as those Judge Greer faced. . . . education could help keep legislators from being engulfed by and carried along with the storm. Citizens would also benefit from and be better able to weather maelstroms like this one with more education about advance directives and the law governing end-of-life decision-making."

In Chapter 5, Jon Eisenberg, a member of the legal team that worked with Ms. Schiavo's husband, Michael, agrees, noting, "The goal is simply to decide how the patient would choose if he or she were able. That goal is most commonly achieved by knowing the patient's *preferences and values*, whether specified in an advance directive or made known to the surrogate in other ways such as conversations about end-of-life choices." Along the way he offers a keen critique of those who seek to obstruct the free exercise of autonomy and personal decision making.

A strong case could be made to support the view that, at ground, the Schiavo case was about *neurology*. One of the nation's leading neurologists, Ronald Cranford, consulted on the Schiavo case and lays out in Chapter 6 the medical facts that should have—but did not always—prevail. "Most Americans know now that Ms. Schiavo was in a permanent vegetative state all along," he writes, "but the conservatives will never be able to concede this medical fact." Dr. Cranford, who died during the preparation of this volume, offers a stinging rebuke to those he saw letting politics and religion get in the way of good medicine.

The case was also about sincere expressions of faith, and Laurie Zoloth explores their practices and paradoxes in Chapter 7: The "description of the shared event of death of the beloved child, the night before liberation, the 'dead one' in every house, is read, of course, in the season of Passover and Easter. Hence, there was no way to separate entirely the apprehension of this death from the apprehension of the approach of the holidays and their rich and multivocal evocations of death and miracle." In the process, she offers a critical view of the bioethics community and *its* practices and paradoxes.

Lawrence Nelson elucidates the criteria for disability, and the use to which it was put in the case, in Chapter 8. Understanding disability is a key to understanding the Schiavo case. When Prof. Nelson observes that "Ms. Schiavo's severe and irreversible brain damage put her beyond disability, beyond suffering physiological or anatomical impairment of function, beyond a decreased ability to engage in typical activities and to have commonly encountered experiences," he is guiding those who hoped she could be counted among the disabled as well as those who knew she was not.

Disability, death, and gender appear in Robin N. Fiore's contribution, in Chapter 9, as among the themes used to frame the Schiavo debate and public perceptions of it. Why do major end-of-life cases mostly (seem to) involve women? Fiore writes: "Our discussion of gender supports the idea that rights of self-sovereignty and bodily integrity are either less tightly bound to the female (perhaps because they are more recent) or that they can be traded off for protection without the same sense of violation that might attach to such a tradeoff in the case of males." Here, "women's status disadvantage" goes far in explaining the social and political course of this and other cases.

Blaming the news media is a great pastime, but genuine media criticism is essential to a free and fair press. In the Schiavo case, the media blew it: "the result was to agitate and inflame public sentiment about the case, based not on truth and fact, but on misimpressions largely fueled by the televised news media's misleading portrayal." Robert Walker and Jay Black dissect what went wrong and offer in Chapter 10 a cautionary tale for those who would presume in the future both to cover such a story and to ensure that ordinary citizens will be adequately informed when such issues touch them.

The overarching goal of the volume is to provide a diverse set of analyses and perspectives, in conjunction with the Schiavo Timeline and other Web-based tools, for those who seek to understand and learn from this sad, dramatic and important case.

NOTES TO CHAPTER 1

1. Much, perhaps too much, in the Schiavo case turned on questions of language use, terminology, and semantics. ("Semantics" is used here in the linguistic and philosophical sense as pertaining to serious questions of meaning, and not about quibbles over terminology. Anyone who uses the phrases or expresses the sentiment "mere semantics" or "only semantics" has misunderstood the terms. We return to language use later in this chapter.) The phrase "permanent vegetative state" is preferred for a person in Ms. Schiavo's condition. "Persistent vegetative state" admits of the possibility of cognitive recovery, which was not possible for Ms. Schiavo. Indeed, to use "persistent" as if it were the preferred term here is in some instances to introduce *by use of the term* a possibility that medical science excludes. If such a possibility were accepted as medically sound and that possibility were to influence decision making at the bedside or in the courtroom, then partisans would by this means shape the facts of the case to win a sociopolitical point—without medical evidence or scientific support. All permanent cases are persistent, but not all persistent cases are permanent. That said, the terms in much discourse and the published literature (including elsewhere in this volume by authors who do not have the intent suggested above) have come to be used interchangeably; we use "PVS" extensively. A beautiful account of the history of terms used to describe various forms of unconsciousness is given by Jennett, B.

The Vegetative State: Medical Facts, Ethical and Legal Dilemmas. Cambridge: Cambridge University Press, 2002. Cf. Clarke, E., and Jacyna, L.S. *Nineteenth-Century Origins of Neuroscientific Concepts.* Berkeley: University of California Press, 1987.

2. The growth of functional magnetic resonance imaging (fMRI) has produced at least one case in which a patient in putative PVS showed brain activity that seemed to resemble activity in normal controls. But all this might mean is that the PVS diagnosis was incorrect. (See Owen, A.M., Coleman, M.R., Boly, M., Davis, M.H., Laureys, S., and Pickard, J.D. Detecting awareness in the vegetative state. *Science* 2006;313:1402. The problem with this single case study is that the patient was recently diagnosed and the authors made unsupported inferences from the appearance of electrical activity to conclusions about "awareness" and cognition. In any event, the patient had intact cortical structures, and so the case does not resemble that of Ms. Schiavo.)

3. For an account of attempts in Florida to broker accord in end-of-life issues, see Goodman, K.W. Persistent legislative state: Law, education, and the well-intentioned healthcare ethics committee. *Healthcare Ethics Committee Forum* 2001;13:32–40.

4. Fuhrman, M. *Silent Witness: The Untold Story of Terri Schiavo's Death.* New York: HarperCollins, 2005.

5. Thompson, J. New Schiavo book offers plots, few answers. *St. Petersburg Times*, June 29, 2005, 1B.

6. Caplan, A.L., McCartney, J.J., and Sisti, D.A., eds. *The Case of Terri Schiavo: Ethics at the End of Life.* Amherst, N.Y.: Prometheus Books, 2006; Eisenberg, J.B. *Using Terri: The Religious Right's Conspiracy to Take Away Our Rights.* New York: HarperCollins, 2005; Gardner, H. *The Church and Terri Schiavo: Living the Truth in a Culture of Death.* Mustang, Okla.: Tate Publishing, 2005; Gibbs, D., and DeMoss, B. *Fighting for Dear Life: The Untold Story of Terri Schiavo and What It Means for All of Us.* Minneapolis, Minn.: Bethany House; Lynne, D. *Terri's Story: The Court-Ordered Death of an American Woman.* Nashville, Tenn.: WND Books, 2005; Schindler, M., Schindler, R., Vitadamo, S.S., and Schindler, B. *A Life That Matters: The Legacy of Terri Schiavo—A Lesson for Us All.* New York: Warner, 2006; Schiavo, M., and Hirsh, M. *Terri: The Truth.* New York: Dutton, 2006.

7. See, e.g., *Layton v. Elder,* 143 F.3d 469 (8th Cir. 1998); and *Matthews v. Jefferson,* 29 F.Supp.2d 525 (W.D. Ark. 1998).

8. Cf., e.g., Calabresi, S.G. The Terri Schiavo case: In defense of the special law enacted by Congress and President Bush. *Northwestern University Law Review* 2006;100:151–170.

9. Tejada-Vera, B., Sutton, P.D. Births, marriages, divorces, and deaths: Provisional data for October 2008. *National vital statistics reports*; vol. 57, no. 17. Hyattsville, MD: National Center for Health Statistics, 2009.

10. This, recall, was partly what the balloon videos were supposed to demonstrate. Also, as Ronald Cranford notes in his contribution to this volume, such reports even included an attorney submitting to Judge Greer a declaration that Ms. Schiavo uttered or emitted the sounds "ahhhhhhh"

and "waaaaaaaa," which were taken to mean "I want to live." Declaration of Barbara J. Weller, Appendix 7 to emergency motion by the Schindlers to have Judge Greer order the PEG tube be reinserted. Available on the Web under the March 26, 2005, Timeline entry at http://www.miami.edu/ethics/schiavo/schiavo_timeline.html.

11. For an excellent and accessible survey (from which the quote from Boethius is taken), see Mahowald, M.B. Person. In W.T. Reich, ed., *Encyclopedia of Bioethics*, Rev. Ed. New York: MacMillan Library Reference, Vol. 4, pp. 1934–1941. Note that many accounts of "personhood" entail if not make clear that a being might be a person but not a human. If rationality is a necessary and sufficient condition for personhood, then a rational non-human alien must be assigned this status. These considerations also influence the debate about the moral status of animals, e.g., the question whether non-human primates are or might be persons will be answered according as they are rational or not. While the "save Terri," anti-abortion, anti-assisted-suicide, anti-stem-cell-research company acquires no small mileage through the simple invocation of a "right to life," there is a noteworthy silence regarding the status of animal life. One should be forgiven for hypothesizing that this is because various scriptures regard animals as appropriate sources of food and labor—this despite the fact that some "right to life" agents go to great pains in public policy debates to identify secular support for their positions. It is unfortunately a common and unremarked-upon form of intellectual dishonesty to hold a faith-based view but to deny it or cloak it, better to attempt to use secular arguments in order to avoid fundamental democratic proscriptions against allowing any particular faith to inform or guide policy.

12. A series of polls during the Schiavo case showed as much, namely that an overwhelming majority of Americans would, if they were in Ms. Schiavo's condition, want the PEG tube removed. See Eisenberg, "Using Terri," pp. 78 ff.

13. The legal reason originates in *Schloendorff v. Society of New York Hospital*, 211 N.Y. 125, 105 N.E. 92 (1915), in which a woman consented to an exam under anesthesia ("an ether examination") and yet refused surgery itself. Surgery was performed anyway, and the patient experienced a number of complications. In the opinion, Justice Benjamin Cardozo wrote, "In the case at hand, the wrong complained of is not merely negligence. It is trespass. Every human being of adult years and sound mind has a right to determine what shall be done with his own body; and a surgeon who performs an operation without his patient's consent commits an assault, for which he is liable in damages." (A number of authorities have pointed out that, strictly speaking, the surgeon was guilty of a battery, not an assault.)

14. This fundamental and simple insight is lost every time a junior clinician is told to "go consent the patient," as if valid consent were something one does to a patient. And it is rendered nugatory every time a surrogate, proxy, or guardian is called in to provide consent without the

contemporaneous authority to refuse. If one cannot refuse, then consent itself, the cornerstone of contemporary bioethics and health law, becomes an exercise in standing on ceremony, a charade played out for the comfort of bystanders.

This discussion of the refusal-request distinction is based on and draws heavily from Bernat, J.L., Gert, B., and Mogielnicki, R.P. Patient refusal of hydration and nutrition. An alternative to physician-assisted suicide or voluntary active euthanasia. *Archives of Internal Medicine* 1993;153:2723–2728, and Gert, B., Culver, C.M., and Clouser, K.D. *Bioethics: A Systematic Approach.* New York: Oxford University Press, 2006, esp. pp. 315ff. Cf. Beauchamp, T.L. Refusals of treatment and requests for death. *Kennedy Institute of Ethics Journal* 1996;6:371–374.

15. The "future discoveries argument" was also the source of some very dark comedy at various points in the Schiavo case: A number of observers suggested that there might actually in the future be a way to regrow Ms. Schiavo's brain—but that it would require the use of embryonic stem cells.

16. Kant, I. *Foundations of the Metaphysics of Morals.* Trans. L.W. Beck. Indianapolis: The Library of Liberal Arts, 1959. This classic of Western philosophy was originally published (as *Grundlegung zur Metaphysik der Sitten*) in 1785.

17. To be sure, conservatives are only Kantians (or Biblical absolutists) some of the time. They become, as they must, staunch utilitarians when planning to shoot down an airplane full of innocent people—that has been hijacked and is being made to crash in a populated place. When cases such as this stopped being hypotheticals, it posed a fundamental philosophical challenge to the "save all life come what may" worldview.

18. I am indebted to Raul de Velasco, M.D., for an exchange that has helped shape my thoughts on this question.

19. Dr. de Velasco notes (in personal communication) that "There are other burdens here and, I think, we have failed to argue this well. The burdens are to the families and society taking care of these patients. Why have we not used these arguments more? I think it is because, deep down, we feel that there is something admirable about the families who make the necessary sacrifices and do it. When you meet some of them it touches you. With respect to the burden on society, the question did not come up much at all in the Schiavo case. I think this is because bringing it up implies two things: first the acceptance of rationing and, second, admission that the fundamentalists framed the issue successfully, making it seem we did not care about the handicapped because we were allowing one of them to starve to death!"

20. Wolfson, J. A Report to Governor Jeb Bush in the Matter of Theresa Marie Schiavo. Dr. Wolfson's report is available under the December 1, 2003, entry on the Timeline at http://www.miami.edu/ethics/schiavo/schiavo_timeline.html.

21. Eisenberg, "Using Terri," p. 96.

22. Colby, W.H. *Long Goodbye: The Deaths of Nancy Cruzan.* Carlsbad, Calif.: Hay House, 2002, p. 380.

23. Horowitz, E. Activist uses Schiavo case in race for state Senate. *Orlando Sentinel*, April 15, 2006. Available at http://www.orlandosentinel.com. Mr. Terry was paid $10,000 for his efforts: "My services were worth the investment. I would have done it for free in a heartbeat" (*St. Petersburg Times*, citing wire services, August 11, 2006. Available at http://www.sptimes.com.). Between Cruzan and Schiavo, Mr. Terry was quoted at an anti-abortion rally Fort Wayne, Indiana: "I want you to just let a wave of intolerance wash over you. I want you to let a wave of hatred wash over you. Yes, hate is good. . . . Our goal is a Christian nation. We have a Biblical duty, we are called by God, to conquer this country. We don't want equal time. We don't want pluralism" (cited by Wikipedia's Wikiquote as a "Sourced" quotation from the *Fort Wayne News Sentinel*, August 16, 1993. Available at http://en.wikiquote.org/wiki/Randall_Terry.

24. The one-page memo is available under the Timeline entry for March 17, 2005, at http://www.miami.edu/ethics/schiavo/schiavo_timeline.html. After initially denying its existence and provenance, Sen. Martinez's staff later admitted to be the source of the memo. See Allen, M. Counsel to GOP Senator wrote memo on Schiavo; Martinez aide who cited upside for party resigns. *The Washington Post*, April 7, 2005, p. A1.

25. Associated Press. Martinez flips on Schiavo. *The Miami Herald*, February 13, 2006, p. 4B. Cf. Bay News 9. Still a hot-button issue. February 15, 2006. Available at http://www.baynews9.com/content.

26. Cf. Colby, "Long Goodbye," p. 391.

27. That the likes of Jesse Jackson and Randall Terry paid visits, and Mel Gibson sent an encouraging fax, is too pretty to be left. Also, while accounts conflict, there was potential in the heated days of March 2005 for a conflict between agents of the Florida Department of Law Enforcement, sent by the Governor to take her from hospice to hospital to reinsert her PEG tube, and local police, whose duty was to enforce Judge Greer's order that she not be moved. "There were two sets of law enforcement officers facing off, waiting for the other to blink," said an official quoted by *The Miami Herald*. "We told them that unless they had the judge with them when they came, they were not going to get in," a local Sheriff's Office source said. But state officials "vigorously denied" that any sort of showdown occurred. Miller, C.M. Plan to seize Schiavo fizzles. *The Miami Herald*, March 26, 2005, p. 1A, 21A.

28. See Harris, J. Is there a coherent social conception of disability? *Journal of Medical Ethics* 2000;26:95–100. Cf. Liachowitz, C.H. *Disability as a Social Construct: Legislative Roots*. Philadelphia: University of Pennsylvania Press, 1988.

29. American Association on Mental Retardation, available at http://www.aamr.org/Policies/faq_mental_retardation.shtml.

30. For a review of some of the issues, and a contrary position, see Balkany, T., Hodges, A.V., Goodman, K.W. Ethics of cochlear implantation in young children. *Otolaryngology—Head and Neck Surgery* 1996;114:748–755.

31. A review of the Website for one well-known organization, Not Dead Yet, reveals a range of counterintuitive, false, and reactionary claims about end-of-life care. See http://www.notdeadyet.org.
32. The text of "Terri's Law" is available under the Timeline entry for October 20, 2003, at http//www.miami.edu/ethics/schiavo/schiavo_timeline.html.
33. Parens, E., and Asch, A. The disability rights critique of prenatal genetic testing: Reflections and recommendations. *Hastings Center Report* 1999;29:S1–S22; and Dolgin, J. The ideological context of the disability rights critique: Where modernity and tradition meet. *Florida State University Law Review* 2003;30:343–361.
34. "Issues surrounding Terri Schindler-Schiavo are disability rights issues, say national disability organizations," available at http://www.ragged-edge-mag.com/schiavostatement.html. The document, echoing those seeking to impeach the credibility of Ms. Schiavo's husband, Michael, says that his reports that Ms. Schiavo would not want to be maintained in a persistent vegetative state should not be believed because "There is just his word."
35. As above, we except Prof. Robinson, whose contribution to this volume makes the case "that the State's compelling interest in the protection of life, if nullified at all, can be nullified only by clear and convincing evidence of the uncoerced wishes of a competent and informed citizen." He also criticizes the very idea of substituted judgment, a cornerstone in ethics and the law regarding the authority of surrogates.
36. In fact, at least according to one analysis, it is conservative Supreme Court justices who are the real activists: "One conclusion our data suggests is that those justices often considered more 'liberal' . . . vote least frequently to overturn Congressional statutes, while those often labeled 'conservative' vote more frequently to do so. At least by this measure (others are possible, of course), the latter group is the most activist." Gewirtz, P., and Golder, C. So who are the activists? *The New York Times,* July 6, 2005, p. A19.
37. For an account of systematic attempts to spin or ignore scientific data on topics such as stem cell research, climate change, evolution, and sex education, see Mooney, C., *The Republican War on Science.* New York: Basic Books, 2005.
38. Stocking, S.H. How journalists deal with scientific uncertainty. In S.M. Friedman, S. Dunwoody and C.L. Rogers, eds., *Communicating Uncertainty: Media Coverage of New and Controversial Science.* Mahwah, N.J.: Lawrence Erlbaum Associates, 1999, p, 27. Other contributions to this volume provide in aggregate a comprehensive overview of the issue. Cf. Hodges, L.W. Cases and commentaries. *Journal of Mass Media Ethics* 2005;21:215–228; this is a collection of brief accounts documenting journalistic failures in coverage of the case.
39. Bernat, J.L., Culver, C.M., and Gert, B. On the definition and criterion of death. *Annals of Internal Medicine* 1981;94: 389–394; Halevy, A., and Brody, B. Brain death: Reconciling definitions, criteria, and tests. *Annals of Internal Medicine* 1993;119:519–525.

40. A definition of irreversible coma. Report of the Ad Hoc Committee of the Harvard Medical School to examine the definition of brain death. *Journal of the American Medical Association* 1968;205:337–40; President's Commission for the Study of Ethical Problems in Medicine and Biomedical and Behavioral Research. *Defining Death: A Report on the Medical, Legal, and Ethical Issues in the Determination of Death*. Washington, D.C.: The Commission, 1981; Uniform Determination of Death Act. 12 Uniform Laws Annotated 320 (1990 Supp).

41. He acted on it as well. On March 20, 2005, President Bush cut short a vacation and boarded Air Force One in Texas to fly to the Capital to sign into law a House-Senate compromise bill "For the relief of the parents of Theresa Marie Schiavo." He signed the document at 1:11 a.m. on March 21. Under the act, "The United States District Court for the Middle District of Florida shall have jurisdiction to hear, determine, and render judgment on a suit or claim by or on behalf of Theresa Marie Schiavo for the alleged violation of any right of Theresa Marie Schiavo under the Constitution or laws of the United States relating to the withholding or withdrawal of food, fluids, or medical treatment necessary to sustain her life."

Later that day, in Tucson, Arizona, Bush said, "Democrats and Republicans in Congress came together last night to give Terri Schiavo's parents another opportunity to save their daughter's life. This is a complex case with serious issues. But in extraordinary circumstances like this, it is wise to always err on the side of life" (CNN. Federal judge weighs Schiavo case: Bush signs law letting parents seek restoration of feeding tube. CNN, Tuesday, March 22, 2005. Available at http://www.cnn.com/2005/LAW/03/21/schiavo/index.html).

At a news conference the next day, Bush said, "This is an extraordinary and sad case, and I believe that in a case such as this, the legislative branch, the executive branch ought to err on the side of life, which we have" (Office of the White House Press Secretary. President meets with President Fox and Prime Minister Martin, March 23, 2005. Available at http://www.whitehouse.gov/news/releases/2005/03/20050323-5.html).

42. Casarett, D., Kapo, J., and Caplan, A. Appropriate use of artificial nutrition and hydration—fundamental principles and recommendations. *New England Journal of Medicine* 2005;353:2607–2612. Cf. Truog, R.D., and Cochrane, T.I. Refusal of hydration and nutrition: Irrelevance of the "artificial" vs "natural" distinction. *Archives of Internal Medicine* 2005;165:2574–2576; and McMahon, M.M., Hurley, D.L., Kamath, P.S., and Mueller, P.S. Medical and ethical aspects of long-term enteral tube feeding. *Mayo Clinic Proceedings* 2005;80:1461–1476. For a history of the technology, see Harkness, L. The history of enteral nutrition therapy: From raw eggs and nasal tubes to purified amino acids and early postoperative jejunal delivery. *Journal of the American Dietetic Association* 2002;102:399–404. For the view that withholding or withdrawing artificial hydration and nutrition is morally impermissible, see the Vatican Congregation for the Doctrine of the Faith's "Responses to Certain Questions of the United States Conference of Catholic Bishops

Concerning Artificial Nutrition and Hydration," available at http://www.vatican.va/roman_curia/congregations/cfaith/documents/rc_con_cfaith_doc_20070801_risposte-usa_en.html.

43. Finucane, T.E., Christmas, C., and Travis, K. Tube feeding in patients with advanced dementia: A review of the evidence. *Journal of the American Medical Association* 1999;282:1365–1370.

44. Nat Hentoff, jazz-critic-turned-apologist for right-to-life extremists, got into the act: "For all the world to see, a 41-year-old woman, who has committed no crime, will die of dehydration and starvation in the longest public execution in American history." (Hentoff, N. Terri Schiavo: Judicial murder. *The Village Voice,* March 29, 2005. Available at http://www.villagevoice.com.)

45. Bernat et al., "Patient refusal." Perhaps paradoxically, Bernat and his colleagues promote the refusal of food or artificial hydration and nutrition as an alternative to assisted suicide because it recognizes the importance of patient control, because it eliminates the role of government in those jurisdictions in which assisted suicide is permitted or contemplated, and because it causes no great discomfort. One would have thought that conservatives would ardently support such an approach.

46. Schwartz, P. Matters of life and death: Patient's wishes, comfort are the main concern. *Indianapolis Star,* April 24, 2005, p. E1. Cf. some of the key points made in "Florida Bioethics Leaders' Analysis of HB701," a document prepared in response to a bill proposing changes to Florida Statutes, available under the March 7, 2005, entry at http://www.miami.edu/ethics/schiavo/schiavo_timeline.html. The measure failed.

47. Clarke and Jacyna, "Nineteenth-Century Origins," p. 315, citing Johann Christian Reil, German physician and physiologist (1759–1813), and his Ueber die Eigenschaften des Ganglien-Systems und sein Verhältniss zum Cerebral-Systeme. *Archiv für die Physiologie* 1807;7:189–254.

48. Address of John Paul II to the Participants in the International Congress on "Life-Sustaining Treatments and Vegetative State: Scientific Advances and Ethical Dilemmas," March, 20, 2004, emphasis in original. Available at http://www.vatican.va/holy_father/john_paul_ii/speeches/2004/march/documents/hf_jp-ii_spe_20040320_congress-fiamc_en.html.

2 ::

At Theresa Schiavo's Bedside:
A Guardian's Role and Reflections

Jay Wolfson

I swam in the waters surrounding Theresa Marie (Terri) Schiavo at the end of her life. The state had appointed me to serve as Ms. Schiavo's special guardian *ad litem*, reporting to Governor Bush and the courts in what was probably the most public death of any private person in history.

Around this unconscious, severely brain-damaged woman gathered powerful political and religious forces. The controversy over Ms. Schiavo's dying elicited the exceptionally active and, I believe, sincere involvement of Florida's Governor, Jeb Bush. He was joined by Florida's Legislature, the Congress of the United States, the President of the United States, the entire civil judicial systems of Florida and the Federal government, and even Pope John Paul II. At least two people offered to pay Ms. Schiavo's husband, Michael, a million dollars or more to abdicate his guardianship powers to her parents, and there were several well-publicized offers to pay for the assassinations of Mr. Schiavo and Florida Circuit Judge George Greer.

National political leaders, some of them well-trained physicians, others successful exterminators, stood before the American people on television and stated that they knew that Ms. Schiavo was conscious, interactive, not suffering from a persistent vegetative state with which she had been diagnosed for 14 years. Even a former California policeman, totally unconnected with the case, wrote a book whose fictitious, unfounded story was published before the state's autopsy report was issued. The politicians tended to speak in a fabulously uninformed, unscientific, and often intentionally distracting manner.

The cases of Karen Ann Quinlan and Nancy Cruzan were supposed to have closed the book on end-of-life decisions and policies. But Schiavo proved this supposition to be wrong.

When I was appointed to serve as Ms. Schiavo's special guardian I was parachuted into a volatile world of personal and political invective. My role was subject to the terms of a law passed in a special session of the Florida Legislature. This law, which became known as "Terri's Law," afforded Governor Bush the authority to re-insert a nutrition and hydration tube that had been withdrawn following a court order. But the law also required that a special guardian *ad litem* be appointed to report to the Governor and the courts and to provide advice about the case's medical and legal issues. My specific written charge was to:

> ... make a report and recommendations to the Governor as to whether the Governor should lift the stay that he previously entered. The report will specifically address the feasibility and value of swallow tests for this ward and the feasibility and value of swallow therapy. Additionally, the report will include a thorough summary of everything that has taken place in the trial court and the appellate court concerning this case.[1]

The "feasibility" and "value" parts of this charge meant that I had to assess the details of the medical and legal history of the case, attending all the while to what, in context, was achievable and had value—for Ms. Schiavo. That was the hook—value not for anybody except Theresa—and this alone created sharp moral and practical challenges. Along the way I dealt directly with Ms. Schiavo's parents, her siblings, and her husband; the Governor and his staff; and the myriad attorneys involved in the case.

My job was to deduce and represent the best interests of Theresa Schiavo. But no written advance directive existed to specify what Theresa's wishes might be. Florida law contains provisions wherein a combination of "substituted judgment" and "best interests" considerations can be applied against an aggressive, objective assessment of the massive legal and clinical record that had been compiled over 13 years.

While Ms. Schiavo resided in a private hospice, dozens of other terminally ill, dying people had their last days there subjected to additional pain, distraction, and, I believe, loss of dignity and privacy. This was because scores of people who never knew Ms. Schiavo were brought to demonstrate outside her hospice. This led to the imposition of intense security measures—which deprived those unnamed, dying, co-residents of the hospice of unfettered access to their families and friends.

Resources of the hospice itself had to be used to pay for a 24-hour law enforcement presence, thus depleting funds that might otherwise have been used for capital improvements or the provision of indigent care. Hundreds of children were taken out of their classrooms in a nearby school because of the congestion and perceived risks associated with the often-hostile crowds gathered daily in the streets surrounding Ms. Schiavo's death bed. Some of the protesters were arrested and charged with trespassing or resisting arrest for trying to enter the hospice to feed and force water into Ms. Schiavo. (Had they succeeded, Theresa would certainly have choked and died.)

Underlying the behavior of many protestors and politicians was a fundamental belief that something was very wrong. So many people with whom I spoke and who sent me messages during my tenure as Ms. Schiavo's special guardian ad litem were desperately confused and concerned about the prospect of her dying by way of "dehydration." Many people said that they would not treat their sick dog or cat that way, and that even convicted murderers are put to death with relative dispatch. Why, then, should Ms. Schiavo and her parents have to endure the perceived horror of a protracted, seemingly painful death? And why should her parents, who love her, not be allowed to take care of her?

Each day in the United States decisions are made to withdraw nutrition and hydration, and families work through the personal trauma and drama surrounding the dying of somebody they love. But the Schiavo matter was different. It evolved into something far beyond Theresa, capturing the interests of those concerned about abortion, Roe v. Wade, right to life and right to die, disabled persons, rights to privacy, and the power of each branch of state and federal government to affect both public policy and private lives.

Through television, the Internet, and an increasingly voyeuristic, virtually engaged population, Ms. Schiavo's manifestly disabled body was displayed partially clad to the world—even on giant public screens in foreign countries. She became a means by which myriad special interests could dress up the Schiavo horse and ride it into town, placing their political or social issue in the saddle. The case was used by false prophets, and it fostered mean-spiritedness even among members of the clergy. It was adorned with misrepresentations and it was such a convergence of political, spiritual, emotional, and intellectual forces that it created a perfect storm.

Theresa Marie Schiavo was thrust into international stardom because it was a new opportunity to deal openly, clearly, and unequivocally with the abortion issue and the moral and political chasm created in the wake of the U.S. Supreme Court's decision in Roe v. Wade that had legalized abortion decades earlier. The emails, phone calls and swarms of conversation, news articles, editorials, and public discussions unambiguously reflected a belief by many that it was time to do more than draw a mere line in the sand. Infanticide in Holland, decisions by the German courts to allow clinicians to make end-of-life decisions that trumped those of family members, and third-trimester abortions in the United States meant, for many, that we had gone too far. For them, the value and sanctity of life had been diluted in favor of specious arguments about quality of life and rhetoric about the allocation of scarce resources. Many sincerely believed that the essential and fundamental values of the American people had been subverted by many years of violent television and movies scored with patently sexual, often abusive, and generally violent music.

No doubt, the prospect at the time of vacancies on the U.S. Supreme Court also fueled the political activism surrounding Ms. Schiavo's dying and its link to the right-to-life movement. With Chief Justice Rehnquist's illness, there was an increasing likelihood that at least one new appointment to the court would be occurring and that President Bush would be making that appointment. The already well-cultivated conservative, fundamentalist political, social, and economic machine was well prepared to activate its considerable moral, political, and economic forces with its sights clearly set on Roe v. Wade.

The remarkably high volume of political and social attention to Ms. Schiavo was, I believe, a reflection of clear and commonly held expressions of an American stew that had been simmering for decades. It was ready to boil. Ms. Schiavo was the main course, and I was asked to inform public policy about the life and intentions of this woman I did not know.

Throughout the period of my guardianship, I struggled to balance tsunami-like emotional and political forces against years of training I had undergone in good science, good medicine, and good law.

I was struck early on by the myth of familiarity that surrounded Ms. Schiavo's tragedy. Everybody in the world, it seemed, called her "Terri," but only a handful of people had ever seen or known Ms. Schiavo. When her husband, Michael, took me to see her for the first time, he approached her and called her "Theresa," fondly and lovingly.

He kissed her and adjusted her head in the pillows. He smiled warmly and stood by her side. He told me about the room, the staff, the police outside who had been hired by the hospice, the list of approved names to see her—and that I was now on that list. I thanked him, even though I would not have needed his permission: I had a court order and was an agent of the state.

The day after my nomination as guardian, Ms. Schiavo's parents, Bob and Mary Schindler, and their attorney, Pat Andersen, objected to my appointment because they claimed I had expressed bias about the case during a TV interview. By suggesting that the case would be subject to Constitutional challenge, they claimed, I had stated a clear bias against the interests of the Schindlers' daughter. They later withdrew that objection and even asked that I be re-appointed to serve Ms. Schiavo's interests.

I sat with Ms. Schiavo in her hospice room for hours at a time. I held her hand, stroked her hair, cradled her head in my arms—stared into her eyes, played music for her, and begged her to help me help her. I was looking for some sign of responsive behavior and not the reflexive actions that characterize the diagnosis of a persistent vegetative state. I applied my health care and legal skills while reading each page of more than 30,000 legal and medical documents assembled over the 14-year history of a battle between the people who loved her most: her husband and her parents—people who once liked each other and who had worked together tirelessly for nearly 4 years in search of hope in a medically hopeless circumstance.

The Schiavo case screamed to me about values and convictions, personal and family decisions, the defining of life and death—but it also spoke volumes about how we as individuals and as a nation make heart-wrenching decisions about the allocation of scarce medical resources. Who will get care? Where will they get it? When should that care be stopped?

The decision-making process in the Schiavo case was not facilitated by ethics committee consultations, and there had been no successful effort to mediate the metastatic dispute between her husband and parents. But decisions about Ms. Schiavo defaulted to the judicial system, and then to the legislative and executive branches of government. I was amazed at the financial resources marshaled and the attention directed to this case by public policy bodies: state and federal legislative and judicial marathons, the costs of one special session of the Florida Legislature, a special session of the U.S. Congress, and President Bush making a special flight from Crawford, Texas, to Washington, D.C., to sign the federal law. While I personally struggled over the profound tragedy affecting the Schindlers and Ms. Schiavo, and the importance of the decision regarding the ending of her life, I was also sensitive to rarely discussed, pragmatic economic issues, including the tens of millions of taxpayer dollars spent to advance and adjudicate the dispute. For Medicare beneficiaries, a dramatic percentage of health care dollars is spent during the last year of life. And in the face of Ms. Schiavo's end-of-life expenses, it would have been perverse not to notice that more than 40 million Americans still do not have health insurance and each day millions go without primary care or essential services, including nutrition.

Who will pay to have tens of thousands of people hooked up to feeding tubes and respirators for years? What kinds of things might ordinary people do to make certain that their intentions about end-of-life decisions are followed?

It is argued that that there is a difference between being alive and living; between existing in a severely, chronically debilitated state, and leading an interactive, enjoyable life; between investing in medical care, pharmaceuticals, and technology to safeguard the future of our society, and spending the same money just because we can. After my review of all of the clinical records and legal documents in Ms. Schiavo's case, I came to believe it was a disservice when some physicians encouraged the Schindlers' hopes. (In some cases these hopes were fostered with patently false claims that experts could literally grow a new brain for their daughter.) The monetary and social costs of medical and scientific misrepresentations in the matter of Theresa Schiavo should not be dismissed. These misrepresentations helped to fuel the legal and media battles.

On the eve of Ms. Schiavo's death, I was leaving the Florida Capitol and encountered an orthodox rabbi standing in the courtyard. He seemed a bit disoriented and had a pile of heavy, winter clothing on the ground next to him. I approached and asked if he needed assistance. He told me that he had come down from New York earlier that day for the express purpose of saving Ms. Schiavo. He had met with members of the Florida Legislature, and was seeking points of leverage by which to get the Governor and/or the Legislature to intervene once again. He argued that a scintilla of life justified hope for all life. Hundreds of people I met, and thousands of messages I received echoed this premise. It was not always just about political opportunism. It was also about genuine and valid beliefs.

Are we hypocrites? Many conservatives made their religious and political positions clear on the issues of life and death surrounding the Schiavo matter: Life must be maintained and preserved, and any effort to allow it to cease is tantamount to suicide or assisted suicide, which we cannot and must not allow. That is a clear and respectable position. But it has been an inconsistent one for some policy makers. Many who "defend life" have remained silent as drastic cuts in Medicare and Medicaid benefits over the past several years have had a greater negative effect on the "culture of life" than the most vocal assisted-suicide advocate.

I was, however, impressed with the responses by so many people to the facts—to the medical, scientific, and legal facts in the case. Once my report to the Governor and the courts was submitted and made public,[2] and after I began speaking publicly about my experience, I consistently received letters, emails, and post-presentation comments from people telling me that they had not previously understood the bleak clinical facts and curious legal details in the case. They asked me why those facts and details had not been more effectively presented in the midst of the public battle. Alas, my job was not to inform or move public opinion, but to serve, at the Governor's request, a single, unconscious human being.

The birth and growth of reality television immediately preceded the emergence of the Schiavo case as a public case, and so it was not particularly striking that the Schiavo saga became a reality show. But the actors on reality TV eventually leave the set and go back to their lives. For the Schiavos and the Schindlers and the millions of others who face end-of-life decisions every day, the decisions made by strangers—judges, legislators, lawyers, journalists—can be transforming, and there is no place to go to escape them.

What if:

- Ms. Schiavo had never have been allowed to die of dehydration, and had, instead, been given over to the care and maintenance of her loving parents?
- She had every right, legally and morally, not to be kept alive for 15 years on a tube without any personal awareness?
- Any decision to not maintain life were the same as assisted suicide?

- It were really cruel and unusual treatment to use technology just to keep a body physically alive, even though the soul and spirit may have long since departed?

The madness of the Schiavo case suggests that all these are correct or acceptable, depending upon one's belief system. It is fabulously relative, not absolute. And my friend and colleague Ken Goodman, the editor of this book, who was one of a handful of close personal counselors during the case, still admonishes me to stop being such a relativist. He contends that some things are just right or wrong, and that my judgment of the personal behavior of the central players in Ms. Schiavo's world is either correct or incorrect.

Robert Miller, a professor at Villanova University School of Law, notes: "Laws authorizing a guardian to starve to death a ward are profoundly immoral, even as applied to those who would have wanted to die; we do not accommodate suicides."[3] This sentiment reflects a strongly held point of view among many Americans, regardless of their political affiliation. Is it any less valid than one that supports inoculation against a virus for which a new vaccine has been created, despite the fact that millions of people may have previously died from that disease? It becomes a question of whether we should do things just because we can rather than because it is the best and right thing to do. But best and right for whom?

It is easy to become another angry voice—angry about the way Ms. Schiavo was treated; shaming the Florida Legislature and the Congress for daring to intervene in the life of a private person and her family. How dare they! How dare Michael Schiavo not tell his in-laws where he stashed the cremated remains of their daughter until she was already buried! How dare he kick them out of the room just before she died after two weeks of being dehydrated! How dare her parents impose any claims against the man she chose to marry, sleep with, have children with! (Yes, have children with; they tried for 18 months, unsuccessfully, and without the knowledge of Ms. Schiavo's parents, to have a child.) How dare the charlatans change Theresa's name from "Schiavo" to "Schindler-Schiavo," a name she never used, to reconnect her to her parents and dilute her connection with her husband?

Who are these people, all of them, to meddle—these parasites of society; these deeply religious people who are prepared to stand up and fight for what they believe to be true; these mean-spirited and selfish people who will push for an agenda of death just because they can;

these champions of personal choice? Yet most of them are normal, reasonable people confounded by the times in which they live, uncertain about what is real and what is virtual, and in some cases, angry and disenfranchised, believing that basic values and goodness have somehow been diluted in a world filled with sex, violence, lies, and terrorists.

The Schiavo case reflects much about our nation at the beginning of the 21st century—as much as it does about a single family's tragedy. It is about a broken society where there are insufficient resources to provide health care for all who need it. While more than $100,000 per year was spent to maintain Ms. Schiavo, health care benefits in the public and the private sectors were being rapaciously cut. The costs of pharmaceuticals, high-tech diagnostics, and interventions continue to increase while accessibility to and availability of health care providers dwindle. There are now communities across the United States without neurosurgeons or obstetricians. The cost of professional medical malpractice insurance has become so high that entire communities face huge gaps in basic health care. Medicare and Medicaid, federal programs that pay for the aged and the poor, are going broke and are being scaled back by Congress and states. Employers are cutting back on health programs they provide. And yet people are living longer and will have increased needs for care, which they might find will be severely limited and rationed. How will decisions be made to allocate scarce, expensive resources?

In this context, the Schiavo experience exasperated many who valued life but sought some balance between principles of individual autonomy, right to life, and the allocation of essential, scarce resources. This is not uncommon. In Texas, a law signed by then-Governor George Bush provided for hospital committees to make decisions to remove artificial life support if a patient's condition were deemed terminal and futile. In December 2005, a 27-year-old, indigent African woman who was dying of cancer had her life support system removed before relatives could visit from her native country. She was medically indigent and had no resources to continue paying for expensive hospital care in Dallas.

I was asked to provide a legal and clinical analysis of Ms. Schiavo's entire case. In the end, my conclusion was that the law was meticulously followed; that the rules of evidence, the rules of civil procedure, and the carefully crafted Florida guardianship statute were thoughtfully and judiciously applied; that the competent, clear, and convincing evidence established that Terri Schiavo was in a persistent vegetative state without hope of recovery; and that her husband's efforts to remove her artificial feeding tube appropriately reflected her intentions and were in her best interests.

Theresa Marie Schiavo died the most public death of any private person in history. Hundreds of millions of people gawked at images of her half-naked body and a recurrent video of Terri's face turning toward her grief-stricken mother broadcast incessantly, internationally over TV. Her face, along with those of her parents, her siblings, her husband, and her husband's attorney, became common, public fare. Web sites were created and remain active where conversations, accusations, postulations, and medical/scientific/legal claims are presented, discussed, and argued at all hours of the day and night.

Unseen and not discussed were images of her as a young girl and adolescent—an obese child with thick glasses; or painful stories of the serious financial problems her parents had endured long before Ms. Schiavo suffered the cardiac arrest that changed all of our lives. Nor did the media give much attention to the relationship she had with her husband: their dreams, expectations, efforts to become pregnant. Equally avoided were references to eating disorders, bulimia and anorexia, and Ms. Schiavo's own life-long struggle with weight.

Now, you might not like the law. You might disagree with how the law defines end-of-life or terminal condition. You might not agree that nutrition and hydration provided by way of a gastric tube is an ordinary medical intervention. You might not believe that Mr. Schiavo should have been permitted to remain his wife's guardian once he initiated an intimate (and child-bearing) relationship with another woman. And you might believe that the rules of evidence and of civil procedure in Florida were inadequate because they allowed for substituted judgment and the introduction of unwritten evidence as the principal bases for reaching the legal determination to remove Ms. Schiavo's feeding and nutrition tube.

But the laws and the rules that governed the judicial management of the controversy were not arbitrarily created. Rather, statutory guidelines regarding end-of-life decisions and definitions and rules of evidence and civil procedure had been carefully and intentionally developed over many years in Florida, where they are similar to those in other states. This is precisely what we hope for when we celebrate the rule of law.

It follows that the one, consistent hero in the horrific Schiavo saga was the judicial system. During more than a decade of intense litigation, hundreds of motions, hearings, appeals, and judgments, the courts stood clearly and conscientiously by the letter of the law.

Moreover, the laws in question were not peculiar—they were not about regulating slavery or ignoring infanticide or promoting racial hygiene. They were garden-variety attempts by an open society to balance respect for life and respect for freedom. In other words, reasonable people could disagree about the morality of any of the decisions made in the Schiavo case. It is precisely for that reason that the role of the courts was so important, and why it was so striking that they agreed with each other repeatedly and over many years.

Put this another way: The upshot in Schiavo was correct just because a valued, tried-and-true process ran its course. (Indeed, Schiavo, the case, enjoyed more court time than most legal disputes since the birth of the United States.) This is why democracy is superior to its alternatives, why the rule of law is superior to the rule of men, and why, every once and a while, it is possible for a citizen like me to be able to participate in and contribute to such an important case—and to help ensure that in the end, what happens is, by virtue of the process, what is right.

NOTES TO CHAPTER 2

1. *In re Schiavo*, No. 90–002908-GD-03 (Fla. Cir. Ct., Pinellas County, Oct. 31, 2003). Available under the October 31, 2003, Timeline entry at http://www. miami.edu/ethics/schiavo/schiavo_timeline.html.
2. Wolfson, J. *A Report to Governor Jeb Bush in the Matter of Theresa Marie Schiavo*, Dec. 1, 2003. Available at the December 1, 2003, Timeline entry at http://www.miami.edu/ethics/schiavo/schiavo_timeline.html.
3. Miller, R. The legal death of Terri Schiavo. *First Things* May 2005, 14–16. Available at http://www.firstthings.com/ftissues/ft0505/opinion/miller. html.

3 ⸬

Schiavo, Privacy, and the Interests of Law

Daniel N. Robinson

The issues arising from the care, prolonged illness, and death of Terri Schindler Schiavo are various and interrelated. Some of these, at the more fundamental level, were either ignored or systematically misunderstood by the cadre of bioethicists, physicians, and lawyers willing, if not eager, to inform the nation by way of sound-bites and fleeting interviews. It is useful at the start to survey just a handful of the issues, not all of equal weight but all deserving more attention than was afforded in the weeks and months of commentary. These include aspects of medical and nursing practice, the nature of guardianship, the status of hearsay in the determination of personal wishes, the level of competence presupposed in granting dispositive status to so-called advance directives, the respective rights and duties of private citizens, the separation of powers granted to the courts and the legislature, and the source and limits of "privacy" and the putative "liberty interests" served by it. The celebrity attained by this case is to be understood, therefore, not solely or even chiefly as a result of the competing claims of spouse and family, but as driven by the recognition that larger and far more significant considerations were at issue.

A single chapter on a subject with such diverse elements must make the most economical use of relevant facts and fundamental issues. Thus, certain details of *Schiavo* must be cited without benefit of full discussion and analysis. Consider, for example, the question of Terri Schiavo's degree of brain pathology in relation to "persistent vegetative state" (PVS) to which so much attention was paid. Entire texts might be composed on such a subject, but for present purposes it is sufficient to cite the statement of Dr. Stephen Nelson, reporting to the Chief Medical Examiner for the 10th Judicial Circuit of Florida. On page 20 of the autopsy report, Dr. Nelson states with commendable brevity and aptness that:

> Neuropathological examination alone of the decedent's brain—or any brain, for that matter, cannot prove or disprove a diagnosis of persistent vegetative state or minimally conscious state.[1]

Accordingly, no attempt will be made to "settle" the question of whether, in light of MRI and related data and clinical judgments, Terri Schiavo was in a PVS, nor will attention be given to the many, credible and even damning facts and allegations arising from Michael Schiavo's conduct before and after the time tragedy entered his wife's life. On the medical side, controversy surrounds both diagnosis and prognosis regarding "persistent vegetative states" based on medical and scientific factors beyond the scope of this chapter.[2] As will become clearer in the balance of the chapter, that controversy would not dispose of issues central to this case.

Given the variety and complexity of the issues, a coherent topical organization is necessary if readers are not to become lost in a welter of seemingly unconnected matters. Choice here is arbitrary but not capricious. What was taken to be the linchpin in *Schiavo* in its ethical and legal projections was the allegedly expressed wishes of Terri Schiavo not to receive the benefit of life-sustaining measures under dire circumstances. The probate court record, as overseen and decided by Judge Greer, reveals inconsistencies in content as well as in standards of evidence. According to Michael Schiavo, he and Ms. Schiavo, along with his brother and his brother's wife, had watched a television program featuring a patient maintained on a ventilator. All three testified that Ms. Schiavo's reaction to the program was to the effect that she would not want her own life preserved in such a manner. Judge Greer admitted this in evidence but was not so influenced by testimony from two of Terri's life-long friends who reported Terri's affirmation of life in the matter of Karen Quinlan.[3] It is notable that the position attributed to Terri by her friends and her parents was based on specific and principled grounds, whereas the contradictory alleged utterance was rather more vague.[4] If, however, she ever expressed either wish, and if her utterances were taken to be on a par with advance directives or "living wills," it is useful to begin with a consideration of such statements and the manner in which guardians and courts should treat them.

There are two main components to be addressed in this connection; first, the nature of that "privacy" right understood to ground the authority of such declared wishes, and, second, the competence presupposed if such wishes are to be taken as informed in relevant respects. Distinct from these two, but necessary if both the right and the presumption of competence are to receive proper weight, is an evidentiary question regarding the validity and authenticity of the avowal. Put simply, what should courts require as proof of the wishes of the party at issue? This question will be addressed below in connection with advance directives and assumptions underlying their authority and credibility. But this and related questions are engaged only in light of the "privacy right" understood to be included centrally among the liberty interests of the individual citizen.

:: Privacy

The issue of privacy within the ambit of constitutional protections remains contested and confused.[5] Giving the opinion in *Griswold,* Justice Douglas recited the now famous assertion that " . . . specific guarantees in the Bill of Rights have penumbras, formed by emanations from those guarantees that help give them life and substance."[6] It is germane to note here that "privacy," from a moral point of view, is a neutral term— that is, it refers neutrally to those venues and conditions of association under which actions take place. It is never sufficient, therefore, in morals or at law, to establish that an activity was done "in private." Law and morals both reach the quality of the act itself before judgments can be made as to whether the venue or the degree of association between (among) participants must be weighed.

The importance assigned to considerations of privacy was highlighted by *Griswold,* but the pedigree is far more venerable. If the sense of the word is drawn from constitutional considerations, one of the more influential early treatises was surely Thomas Cooley's *Treatise of the Law of Torts,* in which the author underscores what he calls "the right to be let alone." Indeed, Cooley was thinking of the insulation citizens should enjoy from intrusive and coercive measures, but consider how he would have "the right to be let alone" understood:

> The right to one's person may be said to be a right of complete immunity: to be let alone. The corresponding duty is, not to inflict an injury, and not, within such proximity as might render it successful, to attempt the infliction of an injury.[7]

Understood in this light, the right to be let alone is one that bars attempts to harm. Whatever might be taken to be the motivation behind the relevant Connecticut statutes, it surely was not to harm either Dr. Griswold or the married couple seeking her assistance.

Cooley's "right to be let alone" was incorporated into an essay of great authority published a decade later, "The Right to Privacy," by Charles Warren and Louis Brandeis.[8] Warren and Brandeis develop the principle or theory of "emanations" not only from express provisions of the Constitution but from far more venerable common law precepts. However, for there to be emanations there must be a source that is itself not an emanation. Warren and Brandeis make this clear at the very outset of their essay:

> That the individual shall have full protection in person and in property is a principle as old as the common law; but it has been found necessary from time to time to define anew the exact nature and extent of such protection. Political, social, and economic changes entail the recognition of new rights, and the common law, in its eternal youth, grows to meet the demands of society. Thus, in very early times, the law gave a remedy only for physical interference with life and property . . . Then the "right to life" served only to protect the subject from battery in its various forms; liberty meant freedom from actual restraint; and the right to property secured to the individual his lands and his cattle. Later, there came a recognition of man's spiritual nature, of his feelings and his intellect. Gradually the scope of these legal rights broadened; and now the right to life has come to mean the right to enjoy life—the right to be let alone, the right to liberty secures the exercise of extensive civil privileges; and the term "property" has grown to comprise every form of possession—intangible, as well as tangible.[9]

The "right to be let alone" would be reframed between the Warren–Brandeis analysis of 1890 and the landmark decision 15 years later in *Lochner v. New York*.[10] The *Lochner* Court was persuaded that the State of New York could not intrude itself to bar the working agreements between bakers and their employers. The baker who is willing to work a 60-hour week was not to be prevented by an over-reaching government by way of arguably compelling "health" laws. The worrisomely protean Fourteenth Amendment now worked to "protect" the liberty interests of persons. The dissenting opinion of Oliver Wendell Holmes in *Lochner* offered a different perspective and one that actually would make firmer contact with the future than was available to the majority of the Court:

> It is settled by various decisions of this court that state constitutions and state laws may regulate life in many ways which we as legislators might think as injudicious, or if you like as tyrannical . . . The liberty of the citizen to do as he likes so long as he does not interfere with the liberty of others to do the same, which has been a shibboleth for some well-known

writers, is interfered with by school laws, by the Postoffice, by every state
or municipal institution which takes his money for purposes thought
desirable, whether he likes it or not. The 14th Amendment does not enact
Mr. Herbert Spencer's *Social Statics*.[11]

Clearly, the constitutional status of "privacy" remains unsettled,
as must be the case. It is something of a distraction to think this status
depends on the outcome of debates between so-called "originalists" and
those who take the Constitution to be rather more elastic and adaptable.
That debate can be traced to the earliest cases addressed by the Court. With
the appearance of the Fourteenth Amendment, the scope of the debate was
widened and, on the matter of privacy, the Court has since been required
to wrestle with it in a varied assortment of contexts. But quite apart from
the constitutional pedigree of the right are questions as to the quality of
actions covered by it. Arguably, the one closest to *Schiavo* is *Cruzan*, decided
by the Court in 1990, and useful to consider here in some detail.[12]

To begin with the most direct question, it may be asked if a person's
liberty interests are such as to protect self-destructive actions. In his
concurring opinion in *Cruzan*, Justice Scalia made clear that:

> American law has always accorded the State the power to prevent, by force
> if necessary, suicide—including suicide by refusing to take appropriate
> measures necessary to preserve one's life; that the point at which life
> becomes "worthless," and the point at which the means necessary to
> preserve it become "extraordinary" or "inappropriate," are neither set forth
> in the Constitution nor known to the nine Justices of this Court any better
> than they are known to nine people picked at random from the Kansas
> City telephone directory; and hence, that even when it is demonstrated
> by clear and convincing evidence that a patient no longer wishes certain
> measures to be taken to preserve her life, it is up to the citizens of Missouri
> to decide, through their elected representatives, whether that wish will be
> honored."[13]

Justice Scalia might have gone further and noted that the common
law precepts fully embraced at the American Founding required the
protection of life during gestation. After ratification of the Constitution,
James Wilson (whose contributions to the Founding were exceeded if
at all only by Madison) presented a series of lectures on law, later published by his son.[14] In the twelfth of his lectures, "The Natural Rights of
Individuals," Wilson first distinguishes between rights that come about
by way of political establishments and those that exist:

> . . . by the immediate gift, or by the unerring law, of our all-wise and all-
> beneficent Creator . . .[15]

Considering next the most fundamental right, that of life itself, Wilson states that:

> With consistency, beautiful and undeviating, human life, from its commencement to its close, is protected by the common law. In the contemplation of law, life begins when the infant is first able to stir in the womb. By the law, life is protected not only from immediate destruction, but from every degree of actual violence, and, in some cases, from every degree of danger.[16]

Whether understood in terms of common law or more specifically in constitutional terms, the principle is the same; viz., it is never sufficient at law to establish no more than the wishes of a private citizen to perform an action or to be its recipient where life itself hangs in the balance. Granting the sincerity of the wishes, further and determinative questions arise as to whether the action is lawful, competently chosen, uncoerced, consistent with relevant State interests, etc. Granting further that there may even be "emanations" judged in *Griswold* to be radiating out from "penumbras," and granting still further that "privacy" is one of these, it remains conjectural as to whether every and any action performed in private enjoys protection under the Fourteenth Amendment.

As far back as *Marbury v. Madison*[17] the Court has made clear that any legislative act that is repugnant to the Constitution is not law, but enactments that protect innocent life are not repugnant to any constitutional provision—or even plausible "emanations" arising therefrom. At issue in *Cruzan* was the balance to be struck between a right to refuse treatment and that recognized and fundamental State interest in the protection of life, even when the source of the threat is the potential victim. Delivering the opinion of the Court, Justice Rehnquist did acknowledge that " . . . the United States Constitution would grant a competent person a constitutionally protected right to refuse lifesaving hydration and nutrition."[18] But there are several other key passages in the opinion that bring into sharp focus the competing claims of the State, to wit:

> Missouri relies on its interest in the protection and preservation of human life, and there can be no gainsaying this interest . . . We do not think a State is required to remain neutral in the face of an informed and voluntary decision by a physically able adult to starve to death . . . But . . . a State has more particular interests at stake. The choice between life and death is a deeply personal decision of obvious and overwhelming finality. We believe Missouri may legitimately seek to safeguard the personal element of this choice through the imposition of heightened evidentiary requirements

. . . And even where family members are present, "there will, of course, be some unfortunate situations in which family members will not act to protect a patient." A State is entitled to guard against potential abuses in such situations . . . In our view, Missouri has permissibly sought to advance these interests through the adoption of a "clear and convincing" standard of proof to govern such proceedings.[19]

It is easy to lose sight of the foundational nature of this interest and thus to fail to comprehend the sense in which so-called compact or contractarian theories of governance are defended. Each person surrenders to the collected will of the governed any number of liberties understood to be available in some abstract "state of nature," in return for which the protection of life and property is taken to be the predominant interest of the collective. It is in the nature of the (implicit) agreement that the individual is no longer entitled to some separate set of arrangements with the State, predicated on eccentricities of taste or passion.

In this light, it is instructive to consult again Justice Scalia's concurring opinion in *Cruzan* on another central point in *Schiavo* and her alleged wishes. Scalia notes that laws prohibiting suicide are indifferent to distinctions between actions and inactions, once the outcome is reasonably certain. Nor is the burden of the offense mitigated by evidence of permanent incapacities. Nor is common law thwarted by the claim that:

> [P]reventing her from effectuating her presumed wish to die requires violation of her bodily integrity. None of these suffices. Suicide was not excused even when committed "to avoid those ills which [persons] had not the fortitude to endure . . . nay, even the lives of criminals condemned to death, are under the protection of the law, equally as the lives of those who are in the full tide of life's enjoyment, and anxious to continue to live." *Blackburn v. State*, 23 Ohio St. 146, 163 (1873) . . .[20]

As for the distinction between action and inaction, Scalia declares that:

> . . . it would not make much sense to say that one may not kill oneself by walking into the sea, but may sit on the beach until submerged by the incoming tide . . . Starving oneself to death is no different from putting a gun to one's temple as far as the common law definition of suicide is concerned . . .[21]

Scalia's position has not become ensconced in constitutional law and perhaps would not enjoy majority support in the current Court. Rather, it does rehearse fundamental precepts of common law in ways that surely have informed the laws of the separate States. More to the point, his opinion in *Cruzan* exposes the weakest points of the privacy-privilege when conflicts arise between the State's compelling interest in the protection of innocent life and rights claimed by individual citizens. Note, also, that, where the State's interest is greatest, so, too, is the evidentiary burden of those who would invoke a liberty interest against it. This was made abundantly clear by Chief Justice Rehnquist in the passages cited above. It is precisely because both the State interest and the liberty interest are at their greatest level of significance that every attempt must be made to establish just what are a patient's free and informed desires.

Applying these considerations to *Schiavo*, the following conclusions are warranted. First, that such "privacy" rights as might be implicit in the Constitution are not without limitation. Second, that the latitude given to the expression of such rights is moderated by other rights and by legitimate State interests. Third, that the State's compelling interest in the protection of life, if nullified at all, can be nullified only by clear and convincing evidence of the uncoerced wishes of a competent and informed citizen.

Before turning to the question of competence, there is that other side of "privacy" considerations, namely the *moral* side. In the current era of a nearly strident legal positivism, one must be cautious before imputing moral ends to law. Theory aside, however, there is no question but that considerations of privacy and autonomy are grounded in extra-legal conceptions of rights, duties, and that common moral sense that the rule of law ignores at its own peril. It is frequently the case, and not surprising, that those reserving to Michael Schiavo the moral right to make final determinations were inclined to pit the police power of the state against the "dignity" of the person, calling for "respect" for one's "autonomy." Citations are not necessary here, for the rhetoric surrounding *Schiavo* was suffused with these terms and their synonyms.

"Autonomy," needless to say, remains at the center of moral philosophy and its historic disputants. It is a term on which rest the competing claims of determinists, voluntarists, and compatibilists.[22] A right of privacy is neither indistinguishable from the faculty or power of autonomy, nor is it the case that any and every denial of a privacy right must be at the expense of autonomy. One is not permitted to inhale cocaine in the privacy of one's residence, but most persons autonomously would forebear from doing so even if the law permitted it. This, of course, was a distinction Locke attempted to clarify by noting the difference between what one is "at liberty" to do and what one does "freely." It is in Ch. 4,

Sec. 22 of his Second Treatise that he contrasts "the *natural liberty*" and "the *liberty of man*, in society," where the latter is:

> . . . under no other legislative power, but that established, by consent, in the common-wealth; nor under the dominion of any will, or restraint of any law, but what that legislative shall enact, according to the trust put in it. Freedom then is . . . to have a standing rule to live by, common to every one of that society, and made by the legislative power erected in it; a liberty to follow my own will in all things, where the rule prescribes not; and not to be subject to the inconstant, uncertain, unknown, arbitrary will of another.[23]

Understood in these terms, one is "free" to the extent that one has "a standing rule to live by, common to every one of that society." Nothing in this tells for or against specific laws that would limit freedom, in a manner common to all. Law in its very etymology *binds* (Lat. *ligare*) and enforces conformity to a rule. To some extent, it might be said that members of society "autonomously" enter into the implicit contract or covenant and exercise their autonomy by accepting the binding constraints of law. However, whether or not the law should respect or oppose the wishes of a citizen or the guardian of a citizen is not to be settled by rather wave-of-the-hand references to "autonomy." In matters such as *Schiavo*, it is the exercise of autonomy and the permissible reach of liberty-interests that are at issue. The questions aroused by such cases must be dealt with, not begged.

Accepting for juridical purposes that the presumption of autonomy under some circumstances is warranted, the circumstances remain to be identified. The "free" actions taken by one who is intoxicated are understood to be *not free* in the morally relevant sense. The "free" actions of a child who puts her name to a lease are understood to be *not free* in either the moral or the legal sense. If, then, one acknowledges some zone of privacy as regards accepting treatment—where both legal and moral concerns center on the right of a person to self-determination—there is still the question of whether *this* person, under *these* conditions has made the determination *freely*, as this very freedom implies *competence*.

:: Competence

Granting the truth and accuracy of Michael Schiavo's testimony, was Terri Schiavo competent in stating the wishes ascribed to her by her husband, his brother, and his brother's wife? If experts in clinical neurology are scarcely unanimous or precise in establishing just what is entailed by the term "persistent vegetative state," it is not to be expected that the ordinary citizen will have anything but a vague sense of its meaning and significance. To say, "If I'm ever in such-and-such a state . . ." may ask too much of one's auditors and may claim too much knowledge for oneself.

In Judge Greer's decision to support Michael Schiavo,[24] the Court understood its sole responsibility as ascertaining the wishes of Terri Schiavo as represented by her husband, her parents, and several other parties. It is on page 5 of the judge's opinion that the case of Karen Quinlan receives attention, for intimate friends of Ms. Schiavo recalled her disagreement with the decision of the Quinlan family to remove life-support measures in that case. Utterly confused as to the chronology of *Quinlan*, Judge Greer discounted this hearsay testimony. The testimony was to the effect that in 1982 Terri recorded her support for the preservation of Karen Quinlan's life. Weighing this, Greer declared that:

> The Court is mystified as to how these present tense verbs would be used some six years after the death of Karen Quinlan.[25]

Of course, Karen Quinlan did not die until 1985, so the dates surrounding Terri Schiavo's comments on the case should not have been at all mystifying. If they were made as specified, they came from a young woman, at least 20 years old, with a history of care and concern for persons with severe handicaps, and with a Roman Catholic background conducing to a special moral attachment to the preservation of life. At a later time and corrected on this point, Greer was nonetheless not persuaded that his error was consequential. Rather, testimony by Michael Schiavo, his brother, and his sister-in-law was given far greater weight and credibility, though their recollections were far less precise.

The failure of Judge Greer to reconsider all the testimony on the basis of this error—which was the Court's error—was misfeasant. In a prosecutorial setting, where liberty-interests are imperiled by imprisonment, an error of this sort would result in a new trial. Consider the following hypothetical:

1. The bank was robbed on June 10, 1982.
2. The defendant was born in 1982.
3. The judge incorrectly reads the birth certificate as establishing 1952 as the birth date and admits testimony placing the defendant at the scene of the robbery.

4. The judge later discovers the error, now recognizing that, at the time of the robbery, the defendant was two days old.
5. The judge insists that there is no reason to review the evidence in the case.

If Greer's recalcitrance on this point was little more than the addition of incompetence to marginal competence, the performance on appeal by Florida's District Court of Appeal for the Second District is no less than alarming.[26] The following are the relevant passages from that Court's ruling:

> . . . The Schindlers argue that the testimony, which was conflicting, was insufficient to support the trial court's decision by clear and convincing evidence. We have reviewed that testimony and conclude that the trial court had sufficient evidence to make this decision. The clear and convincing standard of proof, while very high, permits a decision in the face of inconsistent or conflicting evidence. See *In re Guardianship of Browning*, 543 So.2d at 273. In Browning, we stated:
>> In making this difficult decision, a surrogate decisionmaker should err on the side of life . . . In cases of doubt, we must assume that a patient would choose to defend life in exercising his or her right of privacy. . . .
>
> We reconfirm today that a court's default position must favor life.[27]

This is precisely the position that conforms to the standard cited in *Cruzan* and with the very rationale on which the fundamental life-right depends. Quite strictly, *when in doubt, choose life.* That doubt surrounded the claims by Michael Schiavo and his near relations is obvious from their hearsay testimony. The opposing testimony, reduced in credibility by the Court's own erroneous management of the relevant dates, actually put directly in doubt the allegations of Michael Schiavo. That doubt alone should have found the Appellate Court ruling in favor of the petitioners by its own logic.

Reservations toward such hearsay arise, however, from more than this source, for surely a major source of defensible skepticism arises from the questionable competence of those who would preserve or end life under particular circumstances. In brief, it is *always* in order to be wary of advance directives, living wills, and non-contextual affirmations. Supposing that Terri Schiavo had seen a film covering the Quinlan matter—and supposing further that it would have been her own decision to have her own life supported under such circumstances. What level of comprehension might be expected of her if her wishes were to be regarded as properly informed? Although the initial petition by Joseph Quinlan included the claim of brain death, Karen Quinlan had an essentially normal electroencephalogram and otherwise failed to satisfy the then-accepted criteria of brain death. Initially, life support included a respirator, but her own natural breathing resumed when the respirator was removed. She displayed no cognitive powers of any sort. She was unresponsive to external stimulation, except for incoherent cries and sighs. Her condition was diagnosed as irreversible. On the supposition that Terri Schiavo correctly assessed the description of Karen Quinlan's symptoms and the prognosis, the question still remains open as to whether she was competent to know what it means to be in such a state. This is not a sophistical fine point. Most persons, even young children, have a frame of reference within which to weigh life under prolonged, intense, unrelieved pain. It is only the rare, recovered patient, no longer lost in coma, who might be said to have some comprehension of that seemingly lifeless state of limbo. If, as was reported, Terri Schiavo's position was, "Where there's life, there's hope," then one might plausibly conclude that, in her own case, "limbo" might be no more than a time-out as medical science moves ever closer to some sort of treatment.

Even accepting as a supposition that conflicting testimony finally supported the contention that Ms. Schiavo would not want to be preserved in a vegetative state, she could know no more about that state as an unwilling patient than she did as an allegedly willing patient. The acronym "PVS" refers to a constellation of symptoms, not to a specific disease. Combined with the cerebral atrophy discovered in her MRI data, there is reason to attribute her symptoms to irreversible and profound pathological changes in her brain. Again, however, even if Ms. Schiavo could have foreseen medical descriptions of her condition, she would have been in no position to reach an informed judgment as to the extent of her deficits, their duration, the possibility of future improvements through medication, medical advances, rehabilitation. The specialty of "oracular medicine" is hopelessly undeveloped—and perhaps should remain so.

Judge Greer admitted testimony on these issues from Beverly Tyler, Executive Director of Georgia Health Decisions. She directed a study funded by the Robert Wood Johnson Foundation and designed to sample opinions regarding end-of-life care. Published as *The Quest to Die with Dignity*, the results indicated a general willingness to let go of life when extreme measures and extreme deficits are confronted. No attention was paid to the fact that the Robert Wood Johnson Foundation is among the most generous supporters of the "death with dignity" movement in the United States, contributing tens of millions of dollars to organizations and programs also and aggressively supported by Michael Schiavo's attorney, George Felos.[28] What the Appeals Court did say, however, was that:

> We have considerable doubt that Ms. Tyler's testimony provided much in the way of relevant evidence. She testified about some social science surveys. Apparently most people, even those who favor initial life-supporting medical treatment indicate that they would not wish this treatment to continue indefinitely once their medical condition presented no reasonable basis for a cure.[29]

It is impossible to determine whether Judge Greer or, for that matter, the appellate judges found little of relevance in Beverly Tyler's testimony. Both courts refer to it and both find it relevant enough to cite the major finding. Neither court, however, looked to still other findings leaving little doubt but that, when actually faced with decisions bearing on their mortality, earlier and seemingly firm positions are abandoned. Nor was any attention given to the fact that, in actual practice, physicians faced with difficult decisions either ignore advance directives or put greater weight on other factors. Research more recent than the decisions of the Florida courts adds to an already established trend in this area. Thus, returns from 117 practitioners facing such decisions showed that actual treatment departed from the advance directive in two thirds of the cases.[30] This is not an example of physicians arrogantly disregarding the express wishes of patients. Rather, it is the experienced clinician's recognition that a patient cannot foresee, often far into the future, the complexities and nuances arising from grave conditions. In sum, bypassing the terms of an advance directive implicitly records a lack of confidence in the competence of the person who stated or composed it. Where there is to be any sort of so-called "substituted judgment" at all, one might be as inclined to extend it to the competent physician as to a guardian-spouse whose worrisomely vague recollections regarding his wife's wishes did not rise to the level of working memory until 7 years after the fact.

:: Guardianship, the State, and the Patient's "Best Interests"

It was at once alarming and perplexing to observe the consistency with which members of the bioethics community were of nearly one mind in their support of the courts and of Michael Schiavo's rightful authority as guardian. That there would be such uniform approval of measures designed to cause death by starvation and dehydration was the fulfillment of prophesies emanating from centers of bioethics years earlier. Daniel Callahan, former director of the prestigious Hastings Center, observed as early as 1983 that:

> . . . denial of nutrition, may, in the long run, become the only effective way to make certain that a large number of biologically tenacious patients actually die . . . Given the increasingly large pool of superannuated, chronically ill, physically marginal elderly, it could well become the nontreatment of choice.[31]

Note the main objective, cited without any evidence of regret, let alone horror: The main objective is to unburden the system of tenacious patients by starving or dehydrating them to death. With a perspective of this nature adopted by those who have devoted their professional lives to a consideration of difficult cases, it is perhaps asking too much of judges and the guardians appointed by them to pit their own ethical precepts against the conclusions of the elect.

A group of "fifty-five of the nation's leading bioethicists" filed an *amicus* brief in support of Michael Schiavo's action in Florida's Supreme Court to block Governor Bush's intervention.[32] It is never pleasant to challenge ascriptions of distinction. To do so by way of rebuttal of an actual argument would be no more than an *argumentum ad hominem*. It is sufficient to observe here that few if any of the 55 signatories of the brief would be recognized by scholars in moral philosophy as productive and important contributors to that field, which, of course, is the foundational field for applied ethics. Indeed, what is offered in the brief might have been taken from any number of textbooks in bioethics, which tend to be thick with conclusions and recommendations but rather thin at the level of systematic and critical analysis. There can be no *argumentum ad hominem* where there is no *argument*. The *amicus* brief begins with a statement of the "four 'central values' that arise from the moral traditions of medicine and nursing, and from the ethical, religious and legal traditions of our society."[33] And the source of this summary? Why, the *Hastings Center Guidelines on the Termination of Life Sustaining Treatment and the Care of the Dying*.[34] The four central values cited are (1) beneficence, (2) the integrity of health care professionals, (3) justice, and (4) personal autonomy.

From a moral point of view none of these could stand as "central values" until their modes of expression and resulting effects were specified. Consider the amplification of the value of autonomy:

> We respect human dignity by granting individuals the freedom to make choices in accordance with their own values.[35]

It is patently false that respect for human dignity requires the undeliberated and unevaluated permission to act in accordance with one's own values. The law itself, not to mention moral philosophy, takes cognizance of just those "values" in seeking to judge their worth and such respect as they may deserve. So, too, with "the integrity of health care professionals," who, according to the brief:

> . . . have a right to remain true to their own conscientious moral and religious beliefs.[36]

Moral and religious beliefs can be "conscientious" but entirely unacceptable within a setting established to foster health and well-being. The Santeria express their religious conscientiousness by bloody sacrificial rites performed on animals. Surely members of the sect who also happen to be nurses or doctors could not plausibly claim the right to include Afro-Caribbean magic as part of a therapeutic regimen covered by Blue Cross. The alleged right to remain true to one's moral or religious beliefs is, as with all other rights, bounded by considerations of time and place, statutory constraints, public safety, public decency—the list is long. Failure to address such boundaries directly reduces the bioethicists' "core values" to useless and pious platitudes.

Turning to the duties of surrogates or guardians where patients lack requisite capacity, the brief sets forth the "three models," noting that all three are:

> . . . under the guiding principle that "the surrogate should seek to choose as the patient would if he or she were able."[37]

This, too, is drawn from the Hastings *Guidelines* and, as with the rest, is open to every imaginable abuse. There are choices a deranged or severely disturbed or retarded or addicted patient might make that would be clearly inimical to that patient's interests, of which the attainment or preservation of moral worth must be one. The patient might have had bouts of superstition and delusion, gratified by costly, useless, or even harmful treatments.

The "guiding principle" as stated in the brief includes what is surely an unintended but revealing qualification. Every attempt should be made to find the course of action that would have been chosen by the patient *if he or she were able.* The nature of the requisite ability is not examined but certainly includes more than the power of speech; indeed, that power may not even be necessary. In protecting children, guardians make choices that may go against the *stated* preferences of the child on the grounds that the child would not make such choices if *able* to see their implications and long-range consequences. Deference to the wishes of another becomes reasonable when there is evidence that those wishes are themselves informed by an awareness of the implications and consequences of choices and a rational judgment as to the relative weights to be assigned to all reasonably foreseeable outcomes. Note, then, that the ability that should be presupposed in applying the qualification—*if he or she were able*—is considerable.

As might be expected, the *amicus* brief rises to its greatest rhetorical heights on the wings of "personal autonomy," for:

> No legal right is more important in American society than the right of personal autonomy—each person's "fundamental right to the sole control of his or her person."

The fragment quoted within this passage is not from the U.S. Constitution or the Bill of Rights or the *Federalist,* but from a Florida guardianship case.[38] As with so much of the impressionistic reasoning now featured in judicial proceedings, this passage, too, might have been better placed in an ethics primer giving dangerous solace to uncritical readers. Needless to say, the *Browning* court has no better understanding of "American society" than does one's next-door neighbor, who, if queried on the subject, would surely be less than certain that there is no legal right more important than autonomy. One's neighbor would presumably place the highest premium on being secure in his life and property and in the lives of those closest to him. The basic rights set forth by Madison in the first ten amendments to the U.S. Constitution do not mention and (arguably) do not even envisage "autonomy" as a *right.* It is, instead, a power or capacity, the use of which renders one fit for the judgments of law. When the police power of the State prevents or punishes thefts, assaults, libels, acts of treason, it is neither depreciating nor inflating the importance of autonomy; it is simply recognizing its effects and proportioning punishment to them.

The three "models" advanced by the ethicists are not "models" at all, but a hierarchy of ruling precepts. The first, honoring the patient's autonomy, would have the guardian respect what are understood to be the patient's wishes. The second is really a repetition of this: Where there is no advance directive or living will, the proxy should decide according to the patient's "known preferences and values." Only when neither the first nor the second precept can be discharged is it then open to the surrogate to choose according to the patient's *best interest*.

It should be obvious on its face that, if this hierarchy were widely adopted, there would be no need for surrogates or guardians at all once it was shown that neither the first nor the second "model" was available. If, indeed, there is no advance directive and no basis on which to tell what the patient would choose, then the identification of that patient's "best interest" would presumably fall to the attending medical staff. Ignorant of the wishes and values of another, one who must make decisions can fall back on that most basic and general interest, *the preservation of one's life*. Where this interest is forfeited in behalf of other interests, it is thus forfeited on the basis of desires, beliefs, and values that are, indeed, highly individuated and may therefore trigger model 1 or model 2. But where the beliefs, values, and wishes of another are totally obscured, the only "interest" is the general interest and, as the only interest, it is the *best*. This is surely the rationale on which the maxim *"When in doubt, favor life,"* is based.

In all, then, 55 of the nation's leading authorities in bioethics shed no light and much fog over the guardianship issue in *Schiavo*, though the brief runs on long enough to make clear that a political position was at the foundation of the entire exercise. The brief opposes the Governor's intervention on the grounds that it is "usurping a substituted judgment decision with a political decision."[39] Governmental intervention "usurped" Michael Schiavo's substituted judgment and thus violated Terri Schiavo's autonomy.

If there had been no challenge to Michael Schiavo's substituted judgment, there would have been no basis on which the Governor would intervene in the interest of the patient and of the parties to the dispute. The fact that the relationship between the guardian and the ward in *Schiavo* was spousal would not be sufficient in Florida law to retain the husband as guardian. Section 744.474, Florida Statutes (1999), relevant to this issue sets forth the grounds on which a guardian may be removed. Included among these are (a) failure to discharge his duties;

(b) abuse of his powers; (c) the wasting, embezzlement, or other mismanagement of the ward's property; (d) development of a conflict of interest between the ward and the guardian; (e) a confirmed report made by the Department of Children and Families, which has been uncontested or upheld, that the guardian has abused, neglected, or exploited the ward; and (f) the improper management of the ward's assets.

Any number of facts gathered over the years of court battles in *Schiavo* were reasonably adduced in support of attempts to have Michael Schiavo removed as guardian. Judge Greer's dismissive handling of the facts provided ample grounds on which to challenge his rulings on evidence. Not least among the sources of concern was the patent conflict of interest arising from Michael Schiavo's *de facto* spousal relationship with another woman, including his fathering of a child by that association while legally married to Ms. Schiavo. His squandering of substantial funds on lawyers, funds originally awarded for the care and rehabilitation of Ms. Schiavo, relates to (c) above, as his refusal to permit even the most humane of palliative measures, surely including hydration and exposure to daylight and fresh air, relates to (e) above. On these and related grounds, the government's interest in the case was scarcely an act of "usurpation." Politics is not a four-letter word, and the courts are not the sole branch of government. A State's chief law-enforcement officer has a duty to protect life and property and to ensure that the laws of the State, including those related to health and rehabilitative services, are competently and faithfully discharged. It is reasonable to consider, if not conclude, that the Court's ruling against the Governor was a usurpation, as will be noted again below.

So much deference was paid to Michael Schiavo as a husband—as if this fact alone was supported by common law precepts covering guardianship—that it is not beside the point to examine all too briefly the understanding of guardianship in legal history. Blackstone defines the guardian as "a temporary parent" and understands the relationship between guardian and ward as "the same *pro tempore* as that of a father and child."[40] English common law established one's father or, if he were deceased, one's mother as "guardian by nature." The debts of such understandings are old, extending to Roman law. Justinian's *Institutes* defines guardianship as:

> an authority and power over a free person given and permitted by the civil law in order to protect one whose tender years prevent him defending himself.[41]

Guardianship is an office and, as such, is ultimately answerable to the sovereign authority, which, as *parens patriæ*, has the duty to safeguard the well-being and interests of all under its jurisdiction. In more modern history, this function was assigned to the Courts of Chancery and, to this day, in every State except Louisiana, guardianship law shadows the juridical precepts developed by the Chancery courts of England. The primacy of the local courts in such matters is a settled feature of U.S. law and is clearly expressed in an authoritative and widely cited New York case: The Court has "a controlling and superintending power over all guardians."[42] Note, then, that in cases such as *Schiavo*, there is no presumption of a husband's natural standing or legal standing in the matter of guardianship. Such weight as might be given to spousal standing is for the courts to determine. Were it otherwise, the abusive spouse, threatening the life and squandering the possessions of his wife, would enjoy immunity just in case she were to be legally incompetent.

Deference is owed, therefore, not to spouses or to parents, but to the courts, which have *a controlling and superintending power over all guardians*. There are ample grounds on which to find fault and failure in Judge Greer's probate court, but the Court's authority in such matters is beyond dispute, subject to challenge only on grounds of dereliction or error. That there was both dereliction and error will be patent to close observers of the Court's performance. But to state the main principle yet another way and for emphasis: Criticism of those who challenged Michael Schiavo's standing as guardian on the grounds that he was the spouse and thus a partner in a family unit immune to governmental scrutiny is simply jejune and uninformed.

∷ Separation of Powers and "Hornbook Law"

Under the U.S. Constitution, each of three co-equal branches of government has delegated authority not to be usurped by either of the other two. It is not for the judicial branch to write laws, nor is it for the legislature to try cases except in impeachment proceedings. It is not for the legislature or the judiciary to assume the police power of the executive branch. And, as the Constitution reserves to the individual States and the citizens such powers not expressly granted to the Federal government, the political life of the nation was intended to be regulated largely at the local level. With the Fourteenth Amendment's "equal protection" clause, any number of state and local practices were subjected to constitutional scrutiny. Nonetheless, as early as the Eleventh Amendment (1794) and the expansion of its application in the years following the Civil War, the Supreme Court has understood state sovereignty to be a core constitutional precept, even if honored chiefly in the breach.

Florida's laws as they pertain to *Schiavo* confer jurisdictional authority on circuit courts, including their probate division. Attempts to change venues in *Schiavo*, whatever the ulterior motive might have been, were argued on narrow jurisdictional grounds and, had they succeeded, would have moved the matter to yet another circuit court. If initiatives intended to restore life-supporting measures to Terri Schiavo were to succeed, it soon became clear that legislative action would be required. On October 21, 2003, such action was taken by the Florida Legislature in the form of House Bill 35-E, which came to be known as "Terri's Law." Section 1(1) conferred on Governor Bush " . . . the authority to issue a one-time stay to prevent the withholding of nutrition and hydration from a patient" under specified conditions. These include the absence of an advance directive, a court finding of PVS, and a challenge by a member of the family to any order to withhold food and hydration. The power granted to the Governor was to expire in 15 days.

On May 5, 2004, Judge Baird for the Sixth Circuit declared "Terri's Law" unconstitutional on its face. Relevant portions of the opinion are these:

> Ch.2003–418, Laws of Fla., (occasionally referred to herein as the "Act") is unconstitutional on its face because it is an unconstitutional delegation of legislative power to the Governor and because it unjustifiably authorizes the Governor to summarily deprive Florida citizens of their constitutional right to privacy. In both instances, these are pure questions of law that require no evidentiary support under any conceivable circumstance. A. Unconstitutional Delegation of Legislative Power Art. II, Sec. 3, Fla. Const., provides that "[t]he powers of the state government shall be divided into legislative, executive and judicial branches . . . No person belonging to one branch shall exercise any powers appertaining to either of the other branches unless expressly provided herein. This principle, embedded in both the State and Federal constitutions, that the three branches are to be independent and separate of each other, exemplifies the concept of separation-of-powers . . . It is a safeguard designed precisely to prevent the concentration of power in the hands of one branch . . . The separation-of-powers doctrine "encompasses two fundamental prohibitions. The first is that no branch may encroach upon the powers of another. The second is that no branch may delegate to another branch its constitutionally assigned power." . . . This concept is so fundamental and universally accepted that the Florida Supreme Court considers it "hornbook law."[43]

But is it "hornbook law?" The Florida Constitution does, indeed, acknowledge a right of privacy in Article I, Sec. 23, expressed as " . . . the right to be let alone and free from governmental intrusion into the person's private life . . ."[44] Section 2, however, grants to "all natural persons, female and male alike . . . inalienable rights, among which are the right to enjoy and defend life."[45] Now, as the very legal point at issue was whether or not Terri Schiavo would choose the termination over the preservation of her life, and as doubtful cases must be settled in favor of life, it is plausible to regard Sec. 2 as limiting the reach of Sec. 23 in such cases.

In Article II, Sec. 3, separation of powers is noted and qualified:

> The powers of the state government shall be divided into legislative, executive and judicial branches. No person belonging to one branch shall exercise any powers appertaining to either of the other branches unless expressly provided herein.[46]

No act becomes law in Florida until signed into law by the Governor. Surely this constitutional provision would not be construed as a violation of the separation of powers! Nor does Article III, Sec. 3 seem to be "facially unconstitutional" in conferring on the Governor the power to convene by proclamation a special session of the Legislature, "during which only such legislative business may be transacted as is within the purview of the proclamation." The Governor has the power to adjourn the Legislature *sine die* or indefinitely when the houses cannot agree on a time of adjournment.

Turning to Article IV, Sec. 1, it is instructive to review the powers and duties conferred on the Governor by the Florida Constitution:

> a) The supreme executive power shall be vested in a governor . . . The governor shall take care that the laws be faithfully executed . . . b) The governor may initiate judicial proceedings in the name of the state against any executive or administrative state, county or municipal officer to enforce compliance with any duty or restrain any unauthorized act . . . (c) The governor may request in writing the opinion of the justices of the supreme court as to the interpretation of any portion of this constitution upon any question affecting the governor's executive powers and duties. The justices shall, subject to their rules of procedure, permit interested persons to be heard on the questions presented and shall render their written opinion not earlier than ten days from the filing and docketing of the request, unless in their judgment the delay would cause public injury.[47]

Clearly, Jeb Bush acted within his Constitutional authority in responding to "Terri's Law" with attempted executive action. The question to be settled by something rather more penetrating than "hornbook law" is whether the Legislature itself undertook something "facially unconstitutional" in—writing a law! There is nothing whatever in the Florida Constitution that would prevent the Legislature from enacting a provision, once signed by the Governor, that would require the executive branch to take action on behalf of a citizen of Florida regarded as at risk or as injured by a deprivation of rights. What the Constitution forbids of members of one of the branches is the *exercising of powers* constitutionally reserved to one of the other branches. The courts cannot call out the National Guard, the legislature cannot vote on evidence in a criminal prosecution, and the governor cannot legislate.

All of this is, of course, "hornbook law," but is also not especially helpful as one attempts to tease out the constitutional issues arising from *Schiavo*. In following the directives set forth in "Terri's Law," the Governor did no more than what he was constitutionally empowered and obliged to do. In passing a bill calling for a stay, for the purpose of gathering further and germane information, the Legislature was well within the constitutional framework of legislative power. To see all this more clearly, a hypothetical, only approximately analogous, may shed some light.

Suppose Terri Schiavo had actually written a will, locked it in a safe deposit box, and then suffered her tragic fate. Suppose, further, that she accumulated a substantial fortune in life and that Michael Schiavo and her own family were the most likely beneficiaries. Were she to die intestate, her spouse would be entitled to at least half the fortune, her family to nothing. Under these circumstances, assume further that Mr. Schiavo, his brother, and his sister-in-law recalled hearing Ms. Schiavo say that she wanted her husband to receive all her wealth, whereas friends of hers recall her declaring her parents to be the rightful beneficiaries. Finally, suppose Mr. Schiavo had the key to the safety deposit box but insisted, on grounds of privacy, not to produce it or to disclose the terms of the will. After numerous appeals to the courts by both sides, it dawned on the Legislature that an *ad hoc* remedy was in order. To wit: That the Governor would have *ad hoc* authority, legislatively provided, to take possession of the safety deposit box and to require a further hearing as to its contents.

The point of the analogy is clear: Legislatures are fully within their power to write laws to cover *ad hoc* cases that may involve very few citizens or even just one. The government might require those planning to visit an exotic land to submit to inoculations. Perhaps only one such person applies for the visa and then is paralyzed by the medicine. There would be nothing unusual for Congress to write a special bill awarding damages to a citizen forced by the government to accept medication that resulted in tragic consequences.

There is no need to belabor this point. There was nothing constitutionally suspect in "Terri's Law" owing to its narrow focus and nothing constitutionally suspect in giving Governor Bush the authority to exercise his constitutionally granted authority in prosecuting the laws of Florida, including, in this case, "Terri's Law." If, in fact, the principle of separation of powers had been violated in this case, it was violated by Judge Greer when he blocked the attempt by the Florida Department of Children and Families (DCF) to conduct an investigation to determine whether Ms. Schiavo was the victim of mistreatment or neglect.[48] The Court here interposed itself between the constitutionally delegated authority of the executive branch and the prospective recipient of its protections. It was, perhaps, at this point that the Governor, even at the risk of precipitating a constitutional crisis at the state level, might have simply ordered the police to make the DCF inspection prompt, safe, and thorough.

▪▪ Rethinking the Principles—and the Slogans

In the heated environment of Senate confirmation hearings, candidates for appointment to the Federal courts are often asked the question, "Do you believe privacy to be a constitutionally protected right?" It is permissible to judge this as little more than an appeal to a constituency, for, as stated, the question is simplistic. It has no content either with respect to the putative right or to the range of activities that would be protected. Content might be supplied in this form: "Do you believe that starving a child to death *in private* is constitutionally protected?" Here the answer is easy. "Do you believe that the use of vulgar and defamatory speech in a private domestic argument is constitutionally protected?" is easy in a different way. The law owes no respect to such speech but it does owe respect to the special asylum persons seek to enjoy within their own four walls. What actions under what conditions are at once "private" and then constitutionally protected owing to a respect for privacy are, to put the case economically, a central part of that long debate on where one's individuality confronts lawful limits.

As was observed often when the law was given a chance to be heard during the long season of rulings and appeals in *Schiavo*, there was no respect in which Michael Schiavo had some sort of right, private or otherwise, to cause the death of another by starvation and dehydration.[49] Rather, the question was whether Terri Schiavo had the right to have her alleged wishes fulfilled. In this action, it was not the State opposing the putative "right to refuse treatment"[50] but the conflicting claims of spouse and parents as to Ms. Schiavo's authentic and competently reached wishes.

It would be dangerously reassuring to conclude that matters of this sort are readily averted by the simple act of preparing an advance directive. Such documents, as noted above, are not reliable predictors of what a patient's wishes will be at the time such directives would become operative. They are not routinely consulted by the many medical personnel who might be called upon to provide services over the course of prolonged hospitalization. They are not routinely honored by doctors and nurses even when the contents are known. As for the contents, they cannot be expected to apply across the range and the nuances presented by persons enduring profound life-threatening and life-limiting conditions.

One chapter focusing on a single case must not reach too far beyond the principal factors of that case. In *Schiavo* there was credible testimony refuting the alleged statements reported by Michael Schiavo, his brother, and his sister-in-law. A general principle in this circumstance can be reached and readily defended.

To the extent that the law considers doubtful cases in this area, it consistently calls for a bias in favor of life. Interestingly in *Schiavo*, what "Terri's Law" was to grant to Governor Bush was the power to issue a stay—not unlike the power any governor would have to stay the execution of a convicted criminal. This is an apt model to be applied whenever:

1. An incompetent citizen's life hangs in the balance.
2. The decision that would have been made by that citizen cannot be established beyond *all reasonable doubt*.

3. Persons spousally and familially related to that citizen are in conflict regarding the wishes of the party at risk.
4. The decision that might have been made by the party at risk is one that, in the circumstance, is lawful and seeks ends compatible with traditional moral understandings.

When these conditions obtain, the parties seeking to preserve the life are to enjoy the benefit of doubt and, if not achieving this through action in the courts, may appeal directly to the governor, whose "stay" would then have the force of law.

There are occasions when the laws, the courts, and the rhetoric of an age give posterity a glimpse into those between-the-lines values that actually animate and direct civic life. Future moralists will find in today's slogans regarding "privacy," "pro-choice," "pro-life," and the like evidence that the moral plane has become so deflected that its contents can be seen only under the harsh light of party politics. Candor alone requires one who would write on *Schiavo* to acknowledge that the real agenda had been set by *Roe v. Wade*, whose defenders seek ultimate security in those recently found "privacy" emanations seen to arise from constitutional penumbras. As protections go, this one is especially porous.

Terri Schiavo entered a twilight time in life and remained there for many years. The parents who so loved her continued to see the little girl they knew, the young woman, the eager bride, the worried wife. Less clear is what Michael Schiavo came to see, both before the tragic event and then in the years that followed. Cases such as this are the stuff of drama and, as with all tragedy, they are lessons, warnings, signals. They lead some toward pastoral guidance, others to lawyers and the composition of wills, others to the security felt among like-minded friends and neighbors. As all this proceeds and gives yet another and deeper dimension to life, there remains the fact—the legal, moral, and civic fact—of what the Florida Constitution calls a "natural person," now holding on to a life that can claim little more than a past and an empty future. Here is a natural person whose condition allows us to see just where we set the bar on the value of life. As the bar is raised above the place where Terri Schiavo is sustained, society must address its collective moral conscience and ask candidly whether this is a victory for the right of privacy or a concession to what Daniel Callahan calmly predicted more than 20 years ago when he observed that:

> . . . denial of nutrition, may, in the long run, become the only effective way to make certain that a large number of biologically tenacious patients actually die . . . [51]

1. "Report of Autopsy" by Jon R. Thogmartin, Chief Medical Examiner, District Six, Pasco & Pinellas Counties, June 13, 2005; supporting report of Stephen Nelson, M.D., designated consultant neuropathologist, p. 9. Available under the Timeline entry for June 15, 2005, at http://www.miami.edu/ethics/schiavo/schiavo_timeline.html.

2. Relevant here is Andrews, K., Murphy, L., Munday, R., and Littlewood, C. Misdiagnosis of the vegetative state: retrospective study in a rehabilitation unit. *British Medical Journal* 1996;313:13–16. The investigators found that 17 of 40 PVS patients were misdiagnosed and fully one third displayed recovery during the period of the research. As the investigators note, "The vegetative state needs considerable skill to diagnose, requiring assessment over a period of time; diagnosis cannot be made, even by the most experienced clinician, from a bedside assessment."

3. After an early but abandoned parental decision to terminate tube feeding, Karen Quinlan survived for a decade but was comatose throughout.

4. Testimony in *Schiavo* was inconsistent and controversial on this point. Terri Schiavo's husband, his brother, and his sister-in-law declared that Ms. Schiavo had declared an unwillingness to be kept alive in a way depicted in a television program. Ms. Schiavo's close friends testified unambiguously that she was in full sympathy with the measures taken to keep Karen Quinlan alive.

5. Privacy as such is not among the rights set forth in the body or in the first ten amendments to the Constitution. The opinion in *Griswold*—overturning a Connecticut law prohibiting the use of contraceptives—is often if awkwardly taken to establish privacy as a basic right (*Griswold v. Connecticut* 381 U.S. 479 (1965)).

6. Ibid.

7. Thomas Cooley, *A Treatise on the Law of Torts, Or the Wrongs Which Arise Independent of Contract*. Chicago: Callaghan & Co., Second Edition, 1880.

8. *Harvard Law Review* 1890;4:193–220.

9. Ibid.

10. *Lochner v. New York*. 198 U.S. 45 (1905).

11. Ibid.

12. *Cruzan v. Director*, Missouri Department of Health, 497 U.S. 261, 283 (1990).

13. Ibid.

14. McCloskey, R.G., ed. *The Works of James Wilson* (2 vols.), Cambridge: Harvard University Press, 1967.

15. Ibid, Vol. II, p. 585.

16. Ibid, p. 597.

17. *Marbury v. Madison*, 5 U.S. 137 (1803).

18. *Cruzan v. Director*.

19. Ibid.

20. Ibid.

21. Ibid.

22. For a critical appraisal of the various positions on "autonomy," see Robinson, D.N. *Praise and Blame: Moral Realism and Its Applications.* Princeton, N.J.: Princeton University Press, 2002.

23. John Locke, *Two Treatises of Government* (1689). Edition of 1724, Book II, Ch. 4, Sec. 22.

24. *In re Schiavo*, No. 90–2908-GD-003 (Fla. Cir. Cit., Pinellas County Feb. 11, 2000).

25. Ibid., p. 5.

26. *In re* Schiavo, 780 So. 2d 176 (2nd DCA 2001), *rehearing denied* (Feb. 22, 2001), *review denied*, 789 So. 2d 348 (Fla. 2001).

27. Ibid.

28. For a general history of the movement and a quite generous estimation of its aims and progress, see Hillyard, D., and Dombrink, J. *Dying Right: The Death with Dignity Movement.* New York: Routledge, 2001. George Felos's association with and advocacy of the euthanasia "movement" is a matter of record. Although this need not be taken as impugning Michael Schiavo's testimony regarding his wife's wishes, it does account for the unusual fervor with which all palliating measures were reportedly blocked.

29. *In re Schiavo*, 780 So. 2d 176 (2nd DCA 2001).

30. Hardin, S.B., and Yusufaly, Y.A. Do other factors trump advance directives? *Archives of Internal Medicine* 2004;164:1531–1533.

31. Callahan, D. On feeding the dying. *Hastings Center Report* 1983;13(5): 22.

32. Annas, G.J., Baron, C.H., Bayley, C., et al. Amicus Curiae Brief in Support of Michael Schiavo as Guardian of the Person of Theresa Marie Schiavo. Filed in *Bush v. Schiavo*, No. 04–757, 2004 WL 2790640 ("Bioethicists' Brief").

33. Ibid., p. 12.

34. Bloomington, Ind.: Indiana University Press & The Hastings Center, 1987, pp. 6–7.

35. Bioethicists' Brief, p. 13.

36. Ibid.

37. Ibid.

38. *In re Guardianship of Browning,* 568 So. 2d 4 (Fla. 1990).

39. Bioethicists' Brief, p. 22.

40. Blackstone, W. *Commentaries on the Laws of England.* 4 Vols. Oxford: Clarendon Press, 1765–1769, Book I, xvii.

41. *The Institutes of Justinian.* T.C. Sanders, trans., Book I, Title xiii.1. Chicago: Longmans, 1876. Cited by C.W. Sloane. Guardianship. *The Catholic Encyclopedia,* C.G. Herbermann, et al., eds. New York: The Encyclopedia Press, 1913, Vol. VII, p. 51.

42. *People ex rel. Wilcox v. Wilcox,* 22 Barb 178 (N.Y. Sup. 1854).

43. *Schiavo v. Bush,* No. 03–008212-CI-20 (Fla. Cir. Ct., Pinellas County May 5, 2004). This is the trial court opinion underlying *Bush v. Schiavo,* 885 So. 2d 321 (Fla. 2004), *aff'g* 2004 WL 980028 (Fla. Cir. Ct., Pinellas County May 5, 2004), i.e., Schiavo V. Since hornbooks are primers, "hornbook law" refers to a concept or principle so basic as to require no elaboration or explanation.

44. Fla. Const. Art. I, sec. 23.
45. Ibid, sec. 2.
46. Art. II, sec. 3.
47. Ibid.
48. DCF petitioned the Court on February 23, 2005, and was turned down on February 25, 2005, at which time Judge Greer determined to grant no further stays.
49. There's a point at which semantic precision descends to folly. Depriving sustenance to an extent that threatens life is understood to be a form of "starvation" which may include fluids or may not. "Dehydration," then, is a mode of starvation, not an alternative to it.
50. The right is putative in that the State does reserve the authority to compel acceptance of medications under certain circumstances. The Supreme Court in *Washington v. Harper* 494 U.S. 210 (1990) ruled that the enforced administration of antipsychotic medication was constitutionally permissible where clear danger was a likely alternative.
51. Callahan, "Feeding the Dying," p. 22.

4 ⠿

The *Schiavo* Maelstrom's Potential Impact on the Law of End-of-Life Decision Making

Kathy L. Cerminara

More than 15 years elapsed between the date Theresa Marie Schiavo suffered a cardiac arrest, leaving her in a persistent vegetative state (PVS) because of brain damage, and the date she took her last breath.[1] The conflict between her parents and her husband regarding her medical care lasted for more than 11 of those 15 years. The litigation over her care lasted for more than 6. It is difficult to keep track of the multiple court cases filed in *Schiavo*, let alone to pinpoint the highlights of their many twists and turns. It is possible, however, to trace the way *Schiavo* developed by examining the statutes and cases governing end-of-life decision making in Florida. In addition, it may be possible to predict how *Schiavo* will affect the law of end-of-life decision making, both in Florida and nationally or even internationally. *Schiavo*'s lingering effects will be bitter and may leave important rights of self-determination and privacy battered, much as hurricanes ripping through Florida leave her shores.

This chapter will examine the history of the *Schiavo* cases to determine their implications for the law of end-of-life decision making. Against a background of Florida law, it will explain that, about 3 years into the *Schiavo* litigation, Ms. Schiavo's parents, Mary and Robert Schindler, significantly changed their focus. A relatively straightforward dispute about proxy decision making then metamorphosed into a political furor, and a debate strikingly similar to those undertaken in hospitals every day thrust an intensely personal family crisis into the national spotlight. The history and transformation of the *Schiavo* cases provide direct links to the second part of this chapter, for the long-lasting effects of the cases flow almost exclusively from arguments advanced and actions taken after that transformation. The second part of this chapter will explore how the forces behind the *Schiavo* transformation continue to influence the law of end-of-life decision making for Floridians, citizens of other states, and people around the world.

:: Florida Law on End-of-Life Decision Making

Florida law is quite respectful of self-determination in medical decision making. The Florida Constitution contains an explicit right of privacy, which the Florida Supreme Court has interpreted to include the right of a competent patient in a PVS to authorize withdrawal of medically supplied nutrition and hydration.[2] Many other states lack explicit constitutional rights to privacy, although their courts often rely on federal constitutional rights as sources of their citizens' rights to refuse life-sustaining treatment. In the Florida case described, which involved a woman named Estelle Browning, the Florida Supreme Court set forth a strong foundation upon which later patients, attorneys, and courts could base the ability to make medical decisions of various sorts. Indeed, Florida courts have strongly supported the right to refuse life-sustaining treatment, even before but certainly since *Browning*, and continuing through *Schiavo*.

Moreover, the Florida Legislature, through statutory chapter 765, titled "Advance Health Care Directives," has tried to ensure that patients' rights to refuse life-sustaining treatment will be preserved when those patients become incompetent, or incapable of making medical decisions. Chapter 765 explicitly includes medically supplied artificial nutrition and hydration as a type of "medical treatment" that can be withheld or withdrawn. It also authorizes two types of advance directives: a living will, through which an incompetent patient delineates his or her wishes; and a health care surrogate designation, through which a patient designates another person to make medical decisions in the event of his or her incompetence. It is also possible that some patients will combine the two types of advance directives, thus naming a surrogate decision-maker while also offering some instructions. Both types of advance directives are common and are in use in most other states in the United States.

One way in which Florida differs from most of the country, however, is in terminology. Unlike most states, in Florida it is a *proxy* decision-maker who may make medical decisions for an incapacitated person without having been appointed to do so by the patient (i.e., one who has acquired his or her decision-making authority by operation of law).[3] In other states, those who make medical decisions for incapacitated persons without patient appointment to such a position (again, those who derive their authority from operation of law) are called *surrogates*.[4] In Florida, the term "surrogate" is used to identify a person the patient has appointed to make medical decisions on that patient's behalf.[5]

The advance directive statutes in Florida, on their face—again like those of many other states—are limited somewhat in scope. For example, according to the text of Chapter 765, an incompetent patient's advance directive will not become effective unless the patient is in a "persistent vegetative state," an "end-stage condition," or a "terminal condition," as those terms are defined in the statutes. Similarly, the statutes on their face require proof by clear and convincing evidence—rather than a more lenient proof by a preponderance of the evidence—that a patient in one of those three conditions would have wanted to refuse treatment before treatment may be withheld or withdrawn. Because Florida's right to refuse life-sustaining treatment is grounded in the state Constitution, there exists a strong argument that statutory limitations are unconstitutional, but no case has yet tested these limitations on an incompetent patient's right to direct in advance that life-sustaining medical treatment be withheld or withdrawn.

In the Schiavo case, it is crucial to understand that neither Michael Schiavo nor the Schindlers made a decision about Ms. Schiavo's medical treatment that required the other to protest in court. Under Florida law, a person charged with making decisions for an incompetent patient may either make a decision and allow any dissenting party to approach the court to protest, or may approach the court in advance of making a decision to ask the court to make the decision. In this case, Ms. Schiavo had appointed no surrogate decision-maker before she suffered the cardiac arrest leaving her in a PVS. Michael Schiavo was first on the list of proxy decision-makers for her because he was her judicially appointed guardian.[6] He was also second on the proxy list because of his status as her husband. Yet, in 1998, more than 7 years after Ms. Schiavo had suffered her PVS-inducing cardiac arrest, Michael Schiavo chose not to decide to withdraw her medically supplied nutrition and hydration because he recognized that the Schindlers would protest any decision he made to that effect. Instead, under a procedure specifically approved by the Florida Supreme Court, Mr. Schiavo approached the Florida probate court to ask Judge George Greer to decide whether Ms. Schiavo would have wanted treatment withdrawn. The Schindlers, of course, protested, and it was Judge Greer's decision in the year 2000 that she would have wanted treatment withdrawn that touched off the furor that eventually reverberated around the world.

:: Transformative Forces

One of the most striking characteristics of the *Schiavo* cases was the shift in argumentative focus over the years. Between 1998 and 2001, the Schindlers professed a belief that their son-in-law, Michael Schiavo, was misrepresenting their daughter's wishes. Thereafter, however, in addition to voicing this belief, they also became vanguards of the disability rights movement, in part by arguing that Ms. Schiavo was not in a PVS. This transformation resulted in the *Schiavo* cases playing a different role in the development of the law of end-of-life decision making than they would have played had the Schindlers' focus remained consistent throughout.

Schiavo I and II
When Florida's District Court of Appeal first considered *Schiavo* in 2001, it ruled that the "evidence is overwhelming that Theresa is in a permanent or persistent vegetative state."[7] The parties involved in the case, in which Michael Schiavo sought a determination of whether Ms. Schiavo's medically supplied nutrition and hydration should be withdrawn, were Michael Schiavo and the Schindlers; no one else. The court made a point of stating that persons such as Ms. Schiavo, in PVS, had "cycles of apparent wakefulness and apparent sleep without any cognition or awareness,. . . . often mak[ing] moaning sounds," and that Ms. Schiavo was "in an unconscious, reflexive state." The trial court had briefly referred to Ms. Schiavo's mother's "perceptions" of her daughter's state, indicating that her mother did not believe Ms. Schiavo was in a PVS, but had found "beyond all doubt" that she was in a PVS. Yet there is no indication in the appellate court's judicial opinion that the Schindlers contended on appeal that Ms. Schiavo was in a state other than a PVS. Rather, the court noted three arguments the Schindlers advanced against the removal of Ms. Schiavo's percutaneous endoscopic gastrostomy (PEG) tube. First, they argued that the trial court should have appointed a guardian *ad litem* for this proceeding because Mr. Schiavo would benefit financially

by inheriting his wife's property when she died. The trial court had appointed two previous guardians *ad litem*, but the Schindlers believed that Michael should not serve as decision-maker without an additional guardian ad litem having been appointed to represent their daughter's interests. The court discarded that argument because Mr. Schiavo was not in fact serving as decision-maker during the proceeding in question. Instead, he had asked the trial court to make the decision rather than making it himself because of the controversy between himself and the Schindlers about withdrawal of the PEG tube.

The court characterized the Schindlers' second argument as revolving around the admissibility of evidence in the form of testimony about the results of certain social science surveys targeting people's wishes regarding end-of-life decision-making. The thrust of the Schindlers' argument on this point seemed to have been that the trial judge, having heard this sort of evidence, had made a decision by considering Ms. Schiavo's best interests rather than her wishes. The court ruled that it was "convinced that the trial judge did not give undue weight to this evidence and that the court made a proper surrogate decision rather than a best interests decision."[8] This evidence had nothing to do with whether Terri Schiavo was in a PVS.

The court described the Schindlers' final argument as being that the evidence considered by the trial court, "which was conflicting, was insufficient to support the trial court's decision by clear and convincing evidence."[9] The court ruled, "We have reviewed that testimony and conclude that the trial court had sufficient evidence to make this decision. The clear and convincing standard of proof, while very high, permits a decision in the face of inconsistent evidence."[10] It then discussed Ms. Schiavo's background, upbringing, and prior statements in determining that the trial court had not erred in deciding that she would have wished to refuse the PEG tube. The overall impression from *Schiavo I* is not of parents arguing that their daughter is a disabled person who should be protected but rather is of parents who, while perhaps wishing their daughter were in a different condition, distrust her husband and assert that their daughter would in fact have wanted treatment to continue.

That was early 2001. After the Florida Supreme Court had denied review of the case, Ms. Schiavo's PEG tube was removed on April 24, 2001. The Schindlers, however, had Ms. Schiavo's PEG tube reinserted by filing emergency motions contesting the propriety of Mr. Schiavo's assertion of Ms. Schiavo's wishes. The Florida District Court of Appeal noted that "the Schindlers have not seriously contested the fact that Mrs. Schiavo's brain has suffered major, permanent damage."[11] It also noted that, at trial, a:

> . . . board-certified neurologist who had reviewed a CAT scan of Mrs. Schiavo's brain and an EEG testified that most, if not all, of Mrs. Schiavo's cerebral cortex—the portion of her brain that allows for human cognition and memory—is either totally destroyed or damaged beyond repair. . . . Although it is conceivable that extraordinary treatment might improve some of the motor functions of her brain stem or cerebellum, the Schindlers have presented no medical evidence suggesting that any new treatment could restore to Mrs. Schiavo a level of function within the cerebral cortex that would allow her to understand her perceptions of sight and sound or to communicate or respond cognitively to those perceptions.[12]

It was still true at this stage of the litigation, in mid-2001, that the case involved only the Schindlers and Michael Schiavo, disputing what Terri Schiavo would have wanted.

Schiavo III

The year 2001 would, however, prove to be a turning point. By late that year, the Schindlers had changed their arguments considerably. Through a motion for relief from judgment, first the Schindlers argued again that Mr. Schiavo was untrustworthy and that Ms. Schiavo would not have chosen to have the PEG tube withdrawn.[13] Second, however, they argued:

> that Mrs. Schiavo's medical condition in February 2000 was misrepresented to the trial court and to this court throughout these proceedings. They claim that she is not in a persistent vegetative state. What is more important, they maintain that current accepted medical treatment exists to restore her ability to eat and speak. The initial trial focused on what Mrs. Schiavo would have decided given her current medical condition and not on whether any available medical treatment could improve her condition. The Schindlers argue that in light of this new evidence of additional medical procedures intended to improve her condition, Mrs. Schiavo would now elect to undergo new treatment and would reverse the prior decision to withdraw life-prolonging procedures.[14]

For the first time on appeal, the Schindlers had articulated the argument that would generate a great deal of media attention over the coming years.

While noting "skepticism" about the affidavit submitted indicating that Ms. Schiavo might show some improvement, the court reminded the parties that the issue was "whether there was clear and convincing evidence to support the determination that Mrs. Schiavo would choose to withdraw the life-prolonging procedures." In that regard, the court said, the Schindlers' motion indicated that there might exist "a new treatment that could dramatically improve Mrs. Schiavo's condition and allow her to have cognitive function to the level of speech,"[15] which might affect what Ms. Schiavo would choose. The appellate court determined that further evidence should be taken on that issue. It precisely described the process to undergo on remand (in which a court sends a case back to a lower court), when the trial court would hear evidence on the issue whether "the initial judgment [authorizing the withdrawal of the PEG tube was] no longer equitable."[16] The court cautioned that, on remand, the Schindlers had to "establish that new treatment offers sufficient promise of increased cognitive function in Mrs. Schiavo's cerebral cortex—significantly improving the quality of Mrs. Schiavo's life—so that she herself would elect to undergo this treatment and would reverse the prior decision to withdraw life-prolonging procedures."[17] Although the law had required Michael Schiavo to support the initial judgment, authorizing withdrawal of the PEG tube, by clear and convincing evidence, the Schindlers, on remand, only had to carry their burden by a preponderance of the evidence to succeed in having the judgment lifted.[18]

Post-Schiavo III

That remand order opened the floodgates. At the time of the *Schiavo III* opinion, in the autumn of 2001, those involved in the litigation numbered three: Mr. Schiavo and Mr. and Mrs. Schindler. While only the attorneys for those parties participated in the hearing on remand in late 2002, *amici curiae* (or "friends of the court," persons not actually involved in a dispute but with some interest in advising the court as to the correct outcome) abounded by the time the appeal was decided in mid-2003. Taking part in the appeal that later resulted in the *Schiavo IV* opinion were the parties plus representatives of several special-interest groups, many of which focus on disability rights and related causes. Specifically, the list of *amici curiae* included Professionals for Excellence in Health Care, Inc.; the International Task Force on Euthanasia and Assisted Suicide; the American Catholic Lawyers Association; Not Dead Yet; the American Association of People with Disabilities; the Disability Rights Education and Defense Fund; the Half the Planet Foundation; the Hospice Patients' Alliance; the National Council on Independent Living; the National Spinal Cord Injury Association; Self-Advocates Becoming

Empowered; the World Association of Persons With Disabilities; and the World Institute on Disability.

Moreover, not only had many outside groups become interested in the litigation, but the Schindlers themselves also had changed course. As the Florida District Court of Appeal later noted, the issue with which the trial court actually dealt on remand differed vastly from the issue the appellate court had anticipated the hearing would involve when it remanded the case. The court noted that it had believed that the trial court would be considering "whether new treatment exists which offers such promise of increased cognitive function in Mrs. Schiavo's cerebral cortex that she herself would elect to undergo this treatment and would reverse the prior decision to withdraw life-prolonging procedures."[19] On that issue, however, the Schindlers "presented little testimony."[20] Instead, the Schindlers contended that Ms. Schiavo was not in a PVS. The trial court ruled, and the appellate court concurred, that the Schindlers had failed to prove by a preponderance of the evidence that the original trial court's order, authorizing removal of the PEG tube, was no longer equitable. Ms. Schiavo's PEG tube was again removed.

Thus, between *Schiavo III* and *Schiavo IV*, the vision of their daughter to which the Schindlers acquiesced transformed from that of a person lying in a PVS to that of a person in some other extreme state. Two of the five testifying physicians (the two chosen by the Schindlers) opined that, based on observation of what appeared to be reactions to verbal or physical contact with her mother, Ms. Schiavo was not in fact in a PVS. The appellate court, however, affirmed the trial court judge's opinion, in which he recounted the testimony presented by all five physicians and concluded that "the credible evidence overwhelmingly supports the view that Terri Schiavo remains in a persistent vegetative state."[21]

This is the point at which gale-force winds built. Video clips and still photographs purporting to show Ms. Schiavo's reactions to stimuli appeared on the Terri Schindler-Schiavo Foundation's website. Newspapers and radio and television outlets learned of the case and began to cover it. Supporters asked the Governor of Florida to intervene. Florida legislators received emails, telephone calls, and letters by the thousands. Public perception was of a disabled person who needed care and was being denied it—a person who simply could not stand up for herself to obtain the care she needed. One Florida legislator even described Ms. Schiavo as "a person who just can't say what she wants."[22]

In response to the pressure, Florida's Governor Jeb Bush, who already had called the Legislature into special session to address medical malpractice issues, asked that body to consider the Schiavo matter. The result was "Terri's Law," a bill literally introduced one day and passed into law the next. Examination of the discussion on the floor of the Legislature about Terri's Law reveals that the letters, emails, telephone calls, and media images caused at least some legislators to believe that the bill would protect a "brain-damaged individual" rather than an individual in a PVS.[23] Terri's Law thus authorized Governor Bush to issue an executive order requiring reinsertion of the PEG tube and appointing a guardian ad litem to report back to him on Ms. Schiavo's condition. Later, in the next two regular sessions, a subsequent, less-famous, result of the political pressure from *Schiavo* was the introduction in the Florida Legislature of a bill titled the "Starvation and Dehydration of Persons With Disabilities Prevention Act."

This public relations transformation of *Schiavo* from a matter involving a patient in an acknowledged PVS to one involving a patient with an undetermined condition, accomplished at about the time at which various disability rights and other vitalist groups became involved, had two distinct effects. First, it focused the Florida Legislature on the fact that patients in PVS sometimes appear to be functioning; patients in PVS do not lie passively without opening their eyes or appearing to react. Second, it provided a vehicle for opportunistic use by the disability rights community, wrenching away a private, sorrowful dispute for public exploitation in the name of a larger political purpose.

Disability rights and vitalist activists attempted to fit this case into a narrow category of cases (those involving minimally conscious patients) in which courts have been willing to impose heavy burdens of proof upon surrogate decision-makers attempting to refuse treatment on behalf of patients. Had an argument that Ms. Schiavo was minimally conscious been supported by the facts and proven before the trial court, then perhaps the Florida courts similarly could have been influenced to impose a more strict standard of decision making than that which was employed. Instead, however, before and after the involvement of those activists, multiple fact-finders consistently concluded not only that Ms. Schiavo was in a PVS but also that she would have decided to refuse medically supplied nutrition and hydration if she could. As a consequence, the activists involved in *Schiavo* were forced to rely on the Legislature to accept the notion of discrimination against a minimally conscious disabled person in a case not actually involving a minimally conscious person.

:: Lingering Effects

The *Schiavo* cases and related legislation thus illustrate a progression. The situation began as a relatively commonplace end-of-life dispute between family members of a patient in a PVS who had not left written evidence of her wishes regarding continuation or withdrawal of life-sustaining treatment. Even those arguing that she should continue to receive nutrition and hydration through a PEG tube—her parents—initially acquiesced in the judicial and medical conclusion that she was in a PVS. Over the next 6 years, however, that portrait of Ms. Schiavo morphed into that of a disabled person suffering discrimination because of her disability—an incapacitated person who was being put to death because of that status. The resulting images linger, and people around the world are likely to see several procedural and substantive legal effects of that change in imagery. Undeniably powerful, the images have caused many public policymakers to question some of the most fundamental principles of end-of-life law.

Procedural Issues
Two procedural issues drew the attention of the Florida Legislature in the debates about Terri's Law. These issues are procedural in that they deal with questions of who should make decisions regarding withholding or withdrawing life-sustaining treatment, not what standard for decision making should be used, or what factors should be considered when making such decisions. The first relates to the identity of the person who may serve as decision-maker when a patient has not designated a surrogate. The second concerns the duties a court may assume in end-of-life cases.

Identity of Proxy Decision-Makers. One issue that the Schindlers raised throughout the *Schiavo* proceedings was whether Mr. Schiavo should be disqualified from serving as Ms. Schiavo's guardian, with the power to make decisions regarding withholding or withdrawing of life-sustaining treatment, because he, as her husband, would benefit financially by inhering her property when she died. During the Legislature's discussions of Terri's Law, more than one legislator discussed whether Florida law without exception should prevent persons who might inherit property from a patient upon that patient's death from making decisions regarding withholding or withdrawing life-sustaining treatment.

Florida law, like that in most states in the United States, does not in all cases prevent persons who would inherit property from serving as patients' judicially appointed guardians, as patient-designated health care surrogate decision-makers, as proxies authorized by law to make health care decisions for incapacitated persons, or as attorneys in fact designated to make health care decisions for patients through legal documents known as "durable powers of attorney." Rather, if a financial conflict of interest were alleged and proven in a particular case, then an individual guardian or proxy or surrogate would be disqualified from serving. That is usually the case in state statutory law, for "[c]onflicts of interest will almost always exist in decision-making about life-sustaining treatment."[24] Those persons most likely to benefit financially or otherwise from a person's death are also those most likely to know the patient well enough to know what the patient would have wanted with regard to administration, withholding, maintenance, or withdrawal of life-sustaining treatment. Therefore, "the fact that a surrogate decision-maker may ultimately inherit from the patient should not automatically compel the appointment of a guardian" *ad litem*.[25]

In *Schiavo*, both the courts and at least two guardians ad litem considered allegations that Mr. Schiavo had financial conflicts of interest, but no court ever found that such a conflict of interest existed. Nonetheless, the political battles over Terri's Law blew through Florida's capital with enough force to prompt legislators, unwisely, to consider denying those who would be best informed the ability to make decisions in accordance with patients' wishes. The lingering effects of this legislative near-miss could cause the issue to resurface in Florida and elsewhere.

The "Court as Guardian" Procedure. Most states, including Florida, do not require that courts approve decisions regarding withholding or withdrawing life-sustaining treatment before they are carried out. To require judicial scrutiny of all such private, sorrowful moments would be both intrusive and unnecessary, as many courts have ruled. Florida courts also resemble the courts of most states in their efforts to assure potential litigants that they are "always open to adjudicate legitimate questions" regarding end-of-life decision-making.[26] The Florida Supreme Court in particular has identified two paths by which a case involving such questions could reach court: "First, the surrogate or proxy may choose to present the question to the court for resolution. Second, interested parties may challenge the decision of the proxy or surrogate."[27]

As already discussed, in *Schiavo I*, contrary to the impression given in the media, it was not the case that Mr. Schiavo decided that Ms. Schiavo's PEG tube should be removed, thus forcing the Schindlers to ask a court to stop its removal. Rather, because Mr. Schiavo recognized that he and the Schindlers would disagree about whether to remove her PEG tube, he asked the trial court to serve as decision-maker on the issue of removal. In other words, he approached the court under the first option outlined by the Florida Supreme Court. He and the Schindlers both presented their evidence to the trial court, and that court, "essentially serv[ing] as the ward's guardian,"[28] determined that discontinuing life support was appropriate because it was what Ms. Schiavo would have wanted.

Governor Bush focused heavily on this procedure when arguing in support of Terri's Law. In his unsuccessful petition for review by the United States Supreme Court in the litigation over Terri's Law, Governor Bush alleged (among other things) that the procedure created a "judicial conflict of interest."[29] Seeking to portray Terri's Law as an attempt to remedy this and other conflicts of interest allegedly inherent in the *Schiavo* proceedings, the governor pointed to Florida law on guardianship appointments, which provides that "[n]o judge shall act as guardian . . . except when he or she is related to the ward by blood . . . or has maintained a close relationship with the ward or the ward's family and serves without compensation."[30] Alleging a denial of due process and equal protection for incapacitated persons in Florida, the governor maintained that a court could not "serve in the dual capacity of health-care surrogate and judge."[31] After more than 6 years of litigation, including the appointment of three guardians *ad litem*, multiple appeals and petitions for review, however, it was difficult to argue that the proceedings failed to accord due process to anyone involved, especially Ms. Schiavo.

In the future, however, such an argument could resonate with legislators, even though it has not convinced the courts. With memories fresh from emails, telephone calls, and video clips, and lacking a complete picture of judicial fact-finding in any given case, legislators could yet attempt to build on concerns expressed during the debates on Terri's Law about the "court as guardian" procedure. Were this to occur, it would be an unfortunate example of how the power of images and the force behind their creation can overwhelm common sense and reasonable legal principles.

The reality is that the traditional power accorded to the courts in guardianship matters eliminates concerns that a court cannot act as surrogate. While Governor Bush cited in *Schiavo*, and future legislators might also use, a statute providing that no judge shall be appointed as guardian, the existence of such a statute means absolutely nothing with respect to whether a court may engage in surrogate decision making for a patient. Merely because the Legislature at one time recognized that it made no sense for a judge acting as guardian to submit required guardianship reports to himself or herself as judge does not mean that a judge cannot sift through the evidence of a patient's wishes and determine what the patient would have wanted in terms of end-of-life care.

In fact, that is exactly the procedure engaged in by judges who are approached in the more conventional fashion. In that approach, when someone disagrees with a surrogate's or proxy's determination of what a patient would have wanted done near the end of life, that party challenges the surrogate's or proxy's decision before a judge, who then must determine what the patient would have wanted. To do that, the judge engages in precisely the same decision-making process, hearing precisely the same arguments, as in the procedure followed in *Schiavo*. The difference is that one party has already taken a step (for example, by instructing a doctor to withdraw a PEG tube) that detracts from the goal of achieving what the patient would have wanted by ensuring that the other party not only disagrees but also has become angry because of the step that was taken. The procedure Mr. Schiavo chose simply represents a less contentious way of commencing the same process. Neither poses a conflict of interest for a court.

Should any legislature require the appointment of guardians ad litem for all patients who are the subject of these types of proceedings, or prohibit these types of proceedings altogether, the law of end-of-life decision making would be set back by decades. The law would shift away from encouraging families, when disagreeing about a patient's wishes, to achieve what the patient would have wanted by asking a neutral decision-maker to decide. Instead, it would force such families, who are already making heart-wrenching decisions, to stake out contentious positions even more strongly than any of them may wish. It would unnecessarily force highly adversarial staking out of positions when everyone instead should be focusing on what the patient would have wanted.

Substantive Issues

Additionally, the furor raised by *Schiavo* highlights three substantive issues that are quite likely to surface with increasing frequency in future legislative battles and judicial cases. Questions may arise regarding the substantive standard for decision making that should apply to incapacitated persons who have not left written evidence of their wishes with respect to treatment near the end of life. Moreover, the subjects of (1) withholding or withdrawal of life-sustaining treatment of any kind from patients in PVS and (2) withholding or withdrawal of medically supplied nutrition and hydration from anyone have and will continue to raise difficult issues. Within a few months after Ms. Schiavo's death, in fact, at least one vitalist organization had circulated model legislation addressing withholding or withdrawal of medically supplied nutrition and hydration, and several state legislatures had considered incorporating that model legislation into the laws of their states.[32]

Decision-Making Standards. *Schiavo* highlights a question that has surfaced periodically in the end-of-life decision-making literature for years. When a patient is incapacitated, his or her surrogate or proxy is charged with making health care decisions in accordance with certain decision-making standards. The most commonly used standard is that of substituted judgment. Decision making in accordance with a substituted judgment standard requires the decision-maker to determine what the patient would have wanted had he or she considered the question at hand. Evidence of precisely what the patient would have wanted, in the form of written advance directives or oral statements effectively constituting advance directives, is useful, but it is not required. A decision made pursuant to a substituted judgment standard can be determined by asking what a patient would have wanted, based on the patient's values, beliefs, and attitudes.

When a patient is incapacitated and has left no or virtually no evidence of what he or she would have wanted, however, the question arises whether surrogates can make decisions in accordance with the patient's wishes. Norman Cantor has suggested that in these sorts of cases decision-makers are actually determining a "constructive preference" for the patient—that they are "imputing choices to a formerly competent patient based on what the vast majority of competent persons would want done for themselves in the circumstances at hand."[33]

Indeed, evidence suggests that, although only a small number of persons execute advance directives, a significant percentage of people believe it would be intolerable to exist in a non-communicative state or a state in which they manifest no or little control over their surroundings and cannot recognize or enjoy the company of loved ones. Applying a constructive preference, one could determine that, even if it is difficult to ascertain the wishes of a particular patient, it is likely true that that patient's beliefs will mirror the majority's on the subject of withholding or withdrawal of life-sustaining treatment, at least as long as what is known generally about his or her values, beliefs, and attitudes would support that conclusion.

In *Schiavo I*, the court discussed evidence that was introduced at trial about the beliefs of the majority of persons regarding Ms. Schiavo's state. The Schindlers contended that it was error for the trial court to hear evidence about social science surveys indicating that "most people, even those who favor initial life-supporting medical treatment, indicate that they would not wish this treatment to continue indefinitely once their medical condition presented no reasonable basis for a cure."[34] The appellate court stated that it doubted that such testimony "provided much in the way of relevant evidence" in a substituted judgment case. It also ruled that, although the evidence might have tempted the trial court to make a best-interests decision rather than a decision based on the patient's wishes, it was satisfied from reviewing the record that the trial court had appropriately made a substituted judgment determination—a "proper surrogate decision."[35]

The concept of constructive preference is not unique to academic literature. Since the beginning of litigation over end-of-life decision making, some courts have included in their substituted judgment determinations information about what most people would want to have done in a given situation. The substitution of judgment for an incapacitated person often involves consideration of all sorts of information about factors other than the patient's statements about his or her wishes. Indeed, it must do so, for most people shy away from talking about their wishes, just as they shy away from executing written advance directives. Given all this, considering information about what the majority of citizens would want in a similar situation does not detract from the ultimate inquiry, and may in fact advance it.

Schiavo has obliquely raised this issue of whether decision-makers should be able to use constructive preferences as part of their substituted judgment determinations in deciding whether to authorize withholding or withdrawing life-sustaining treatment. In most cases and in most states, decision-makers must use the substituted judgment standard if evidence of a patient's wishes is available, rather than discarding it entirely for a constructive preference standard. Evidence regarding the majority's preferences can be and ought to be considered as part of the decision-making process when determining what a patient's wishes would have been. The Florida Supreme Court did not rule on the issue in *Schiavo,* and it could resurface, especially as legislators nationwide recall how Florida policymakers were buffeted by the force of the disability rights and vitalist movements in *Schiavo.*

Patients in PVS. Terri Schiavo was in a PVS. So was Nancy Cruzan. [36] So was Karen Ann Quinlan.[37] So were the patients about whom most of the reported end-of-life decision-making appellate cases in the United States have been litigated. Patients in PVS, like patients receiving medically supplied nutrition and hydration (and often they are the same), present emotionally difficult cases.

These cases are difficult because, as noted by the *Schiavo* courts, patients in PVS do not always look as if they lack cognitive functioning. They do not necessarily appear to the casual observer to lack cognitive function, and they certainly do not appear that way to loving family members. The Florida Legislature was shocked to learn that a patient in a PVS occasionally can appear awake, and can even seem to react to certain stimuli. One legislator later even stated that "this was not a PVS in terms of what we meant" at the time of a statutory revision in 1999.[38] It seems not to be a far stretch to imagine that various state legislators may, in the aftermath of *Schiavo,* revisit their statutory descriptions of patients in PVS or, most dangerously, debate whether to permit persons to refuse treatment when in PVS. That would be unconstitutional under a Florida Supreme Court precedent ruling that a person in a PVS had a constitutional right to the withdrawal of medically supplied nutrition and hydration. It similarly would be suspect in other states.

Such a move also would be unfortunate, if not tragic, because PVS patients are cognitively unaware. They have no higher brain function even though they make sounds, appear to react, and display other confusing signs. They lack the awareness that most of us want and value up until the time we die. Most people do not want to exist in PVS. The law must permit these patients to refuse treatment, especially invasive treatment such as surgically implanted sources of artificial nutrition and hydration.

Medically Supplied Nutrition and Hydration. Withholding or withdrawing medically supplied nutrition and hydration always has been a sensitive issue. The only United States Supreme Court case addressing a withholding and withdrawal of treatment issue, *Cruzan v. Director, Missouri Department of Health,* involved the requested withdrawal of medically supplied nutrition and hydration. As of the beginning of 2005, courts and state attorneys general had issued more than 60 reported opinions concerning withholding or withdrawing of medically supplied nutrition and hydration.[39] The issue is more difficult than those regarding other forms of medical treatment because a person suggesting to family members that withdrawal of medically supplied nutrition and hydration is appropriate, often sounds, to those family members, as if he or she is saying, "Don't *feed* this person or give her water." *Schiavo* has triggered an attempt at legal retrenchment from the firmly established ethical view that medically supplied nutrition and hydration is medical treatment that can be withheld or withdrawn on the same basis as other life-sustaining medical treatments.

At least in the minds of some persons of the Roman Catholic faith, the issue of withholding or withdrawing medically supplied nutrition and hydration became more debatable in 2004, as *Schiavo* was being argued, than previously. There always had been some level of discomfort with withholding or withdrawing medically supplied nutrition and hydration among some Roman Catholics. Until a 2004 statement by Pope John Paul II, however, it had been clear that the Church's position was that it was appropriate to determine on a case-by-case basis, based on a burden–benefit analysis, whether to require administration of medically supplied nutrition and hydration. In other words, medically supplied nutrition and hydration, in the Catholic tradition, constituted the sort of treatment that could be withheld or withdrawn under much the same analysis as other life-sustaining medical treatments. In 2004, however, addressing the International Congress on "Life-Sustaining Treatments and Vegetative State: Scientific Advances and Ethical Dilemmas," the Pope stated that "the administration of water and food, even when provided by artificial means, always represents a natural means of preserving life, not a medical act," and "should be considered, in principle, ordinary and proportionate, and as such morally obligatory."[40]

The Pope's statement combined with *Schiavo* itself to ensure that withholding or withdrawal of medically supplied nutrition and hydration will remain a hot topic in the realm of end-of-life decision making. Individual religious Catholics are free to consider the Pope's statement as instructive even if it is not binding on Catholic institutions or the American Church. Religiously motivated voters are an important part of politicians' constituencies, as demonstrated by the results of the 2004 presidential election. Many voters, religiously motivated or not, contact their legislators on issues that are important to them, as many did in *Schiavo*, and the Pope's statement will cause many religiously motivated voters to believe the issue is important. If a legislature is already queasy about withholding or withdrawing medically supplied nutrition and hydration, as was the Florida Legislature, hearing constituent vocalization could indeed trigger special legislative treatment.

Some statutes in various states support this conclusion, as did the introduction of model legislation titled the "Starvation and Dehydration of Persons With Disabilities Prevention Act" in various legislatures during and after *Schiavo*. The promulgation of such legislation, as well as its consideration by several states, illustrates the power of the *Schiavo* story. What began as an everyday end-of-life decision-making dispute became distinctive through legal and visual manipulation, and has reverberated in several state legislatures by virtue of exploitation by a powerful interest group.

The evolution of existing state law provides some lessons. At one time, many statutes prohibited the forgoing of medically supplied nutrition and hydration pursuant to statutory advance directives. In 1990, in *Cruzan*, a majority of the justices on the United States Supreme Court opined (although not in one consolidated, majority opinion) that medically supplied nutrition and hydration constitutes a form of medical treatment. Most state statutes, falling in line with that conclusion, now permit its withholding or withdrawal. Some states, however, impose special requirements before it can be withheld or withdrawn in accordance with written directives. For example, in a handful of states, when a written advance directive is involved, "nutrition and hydration may be withheld only if the principal has specifically refused them or the principal's wishes regarding them are reasonably known or can, with reasonable diligence, be ascertained."[41] Such statutes govern only a small percentage of actual instances of withholding and withdrawing, since most withholding and withdrawing takes place in the absence of a written advance directive. They do, however, illustrate the point: Emotional baggage accompanying the withholding or withdrawing of medically supplied nutrition and hydration sometimes causes it to be viewed differently from other forms of life-sustaining treatment.

Through its very name, the model Starvation and Dehydration of Persons With Disabilities Prevention Act clearly played on the emotions surrounding withholding or withdrawing medically supplied nutrition and hydration. The title of this act was designed to incite emotions and create an image of a healthy person wasting away, in a condition that many people associate with great pain, although research demonstrates that unmanageable suffering is not involved, and a "lack of hydration and nutrition . . . may even have an analgesic effect."[42] Even though, as a technical matter, a body deprived of artificial nutrition and hydration eventually will cease functioning because of lack of fuel, or, more likely, lack of fluids, it is not the discontinuation of the medical procedure that causes the cessation of functioning. Instead, it is the condition of the patient that makes it impossible for that patient to receive nutrition or hydration through other than a medical procedure involving bodily invasion. Refraining from using technical medical procedures to take over when the body itself cannot perform functions on its own is at the core of the right to refuse treatment. It is the same as turning off a respirator when the body cannot breathe on its own; it constitutes removal of a mechanical way of providing a function the body can no longer perform on its own. Yet the title of the model act reinforces, in a dramatic way, the impression that medically supplied nutrition and hydration differs greatly from other forms of medical treatment.

Even more crucially, the Starvation and Dehydration of Persons With Disabilities Prevention Act, introduced in the Florida Legislature and many other state legislatures during 2005,[43] would prevent the vast majority of persons from exercising their right to self-determination. The model law would distinguish medically supplied nutrition and hydration from all other types of medical treatment. It then would establish a presumption against the refusal of such an intervention, contrary to established case law in many state courts and the United States Supreme Court that medically supplied nutrition and hydration does not stand in a class by itself but rather is a form of medical treatment representing exactly the sort of invasive procedure that all persons in the United States, under both the common law and state and federal constitutions, may refuse. Moreover, in addition to establishing a presumption that infringes upon patients' rights in the first instance, the model law would permit that presumption to be overridden only in the most unlikely of circumstances: (1) when, in reasonable medical judgment (a defined term), provision of medically supplied nutrition and hydration is "not medically possible," "would hasten death," or "would not contribute to sustaining the person's life;" (2)

when the patient has executed a written advance directive specifically authorizing the withholding or withdrawing of medically supplied nutrition and hydration; or (3) when there exists clear and convincing evidence that the patient gave prior express, informed consent relating to the currently existing circumstances and treatment alternatives (a virtual impossibility to achieve).[44] It thus would permit withholding or withdrawing nutrition and hydration in only three instances, which, even collectively, could apply to such a small number of cases that the statute essentially would establish an irrebuttable presumption against the refusal of medically supplied nutrition and hydration.

Internationally, too, *Schiavo's* effects continue to reverberate in bodies considering end-of-life decision-making issues. Within 8 months of Ms. Schiavo's death, the Italian National Committee on Bioethics, apparently influenced by both the Pope's statement and the *Schiavo* cases, opined that medically supplied nutrition and hydration should not be considered medical treatment and should not be withheld or withdrawn, even when a patient requested withholding or withdrawal in a written advance directive. It is not unlikely that other heavily Roman Catholic countries will react in the same way.

In sum, the imagery accompanying the *Schiavo* cases and the strength of the forces propelling them have combined powerfully with the religious overtones and emotional resonance of the nutrition and hydration issue. At the time of the passage of Terri's Law, the Florida House and Senate floors were filled with legislators referring to "starvation" and to the common misconception that withdrawal of medically supplied nutrition and hydration causes pain or suffering. Medically supplied nutrition and hydration has always engendered more emotional responses than other life-sustaining medical treatments, and so legislative efforts to distinguish between it and all the other life-sustaining treatments will continue to cloud the horizon.

∷ Conclusion

The waves kicked up by the *Schiavo* storm will continue to ebb and flow. Images of Ms. Schiavo as she was portrayed after the transformation in litigation strategy described here will overshadow the law of end-of-life decision making for years. The *Schiavo* cases may increase pressure on policymakers to change laws about guardianship qualifications, judicial procedures, decision-making standards, patients in PVS, or medically supplied nutrition and hydration. While being buffeted by forces such as those behind the *Schiavo* cases, legislators, courts, and other policymakers must be careful not to destroy citizens' rights of self-determination or to allow their liberty interests to be eroded.

Practical consequences accompany such potential legal effects. Politically, one must contemplate what Terri's Law did to citizens' feelings about the legislative process. The forces propelling *Schiavo* have capitalized on this opportunity to demonstrate that legislators and governors concerned about re-election cannot consider end-of-life decision making an area of settled consensus. Citizens are unlikely to be left with a good impression of the way that government works after hearing a governor and legislature, in responding to politically powerful forces, state (as in *Schiavo*) that they do not care whether a statute is constitutional if they believe that it represents an attempt to achieve a good result. Politics also inevitably reach into the judicial system where judges are elected, and another practical outcome of *Schiavo* may be increased judicial reluctance to deal with end-of-life decision making. It is difficult to imagine a judge wanting to be in the position of Pinellas Circuit Court Judge George Greer, who handled most of the trial-court-level proceedings and who endured several motions to recuse and other allegations of bias during the years of the *Schiavo* litigation. It similarly is difficult to imagine a judge who would want to face a retention election (as Judge Greer did, victoriously) knowing that others are willing to run in opposition because of rulings in these types of cases.

More education in the law of end-of-life decision making would help lessen some of these practical effects on judges, legislators, and the citizenry. On the judicial front, more education would help judges feel prepared to hear cases and to produce considered results even in the face of heated reactions such as those Judge Greer faced. On the legislative front, education could help keep legislators from being engulfed by and carried along with the storm. Citizens would also benefit from and be better able to weather maelstroms like this one with more education about advance directives and the law governing end-of-life decision making. No matter what position they take on refusal of life-sustaining treatment, one message people have read or otherwise internalized from *Schiavo* is that they should memorialize their wishes regarding end-of-life decision making. Although an increase in advance directives may present the medical and legal communities with additional challenges in the future, their execution would be a positive result of this tragic commingling of strong political winds with two parents' wishes for their neurologically devastated daughter.

1. This chapter is adapted with permission from Kathy L. Cerminara, Tracking the storm: The far-reaching power of the forces propelling the Schiavo cases. *Stetson Law Review* 2005;35:147–178.
2. Fla. Const. Art. I, sec. 23; *In re Browning*, 568 So. 2d 4 (Fla. 1990).
3. See Fla. Stat. ch. 765.401 (2004).
4. See Meisel, A., and Cerminara, K.L. *The Right to Die: The Law of End-of-Life Decisionmaking.* New York: Aspen, 3rd ed., 2004, 7.01[B][4], [6]
5. See Fla. Stat. ch. 765.205 (2004).
6. Fla. Stat. ch. 765.401 (2004).
7. *In re Schiavo*, 780 So. 2d 176, 177 (Fla. Dist. Ct. App. 2001), review denied 789 So. 2d 348 (Fla. 2001) (Schiavo I); available under the Timeline entry for January 24, 2001, at http://www.miami.edu/ethics/schiavo/schiavo_timeline.html. The law uses the term "persistent vegetative state," although neurologists will differentiate between a "persistent" and a "permanent" vegetative state. Roughly speaking, a patient is said to be in a persistent vegetative state when in a "cognitively unresponsive state" for more than a month and to be in a permanent vegetative state if the condition lasts for 12 months. Childs, N.L., and Mercer, W.N. Late improvement in consciousness after post-traumatic vegetative state. *New England Journal of Medicine* 1996;334:24–25.
8. Schiavo I, 780 So. 2d at 179.
9. Ibid.
10. Ibid. (citing *Browning*, 543 So. 2d at 273).
11. *In re Schiavo*, 792 So. 2d 551, 560 (Fla. Dist. Ct. App. 2001) (Schiavo II); available under the Timeline under for July 11, 2001, at http://www.miami.edu/ethics/schiavo/schiavo_timeline.html.
12. Ibid. (emphasis added).
13. *In re Schiavo*, 800 So. 2d 640, 643 (Fla. Dist. Ct. App. 2001) (Schiavo III); available under the Timeline under for October 17, 2001, at http://www.miami.edu/ethics/schiavo/schiavo_timeline.html.
14. Schiavo III, 800 So. 2d at 643–644.
15. Schiavo III, 800 So. 2d at 645.
16. Ibid.
17. Ibid.
18. Ibid.
19. Schiavo IV, 851 So. 2d at 185.
20. Ibid.
21. *In re Schiavo*, 2002 WL 31817960, *2-*3 (Fla. Cir. Ct. Nov. 22, 2002) (commenting at *3 that "[e]ven Dr. Maxfield [who was testifying for the Schindlers] acknowledges that vegetative patients can track on occasion and that smiling can be a reflex."); available under the Timeline entry for November 22, 2002, at http://www.miami.edu/ethics/schiavo/schiavo_timeline.html.
22. Audio tape, Fla. H.R. Spec. Sess. E HB35-E (October 20, 2003).

23. Audio tape: Fla. H.R. Spec. Sess. E HB35-E at 1:00+. While it is not incorrect to term an individual in a PVS a "brain-damaged individual," use of that sort of language raises a different image than does use of the term "PVS."

24. See "The Right to Die," ' 3.24[C]] at 3–96 (citing *Cruzan v. Director*, Mo. Dep't of Health, 497 U.S. 261, 286 (1990)).

25. Schiavo I, 780 So. 2d at 178.

26. *Browning*, 568 So. 2d at 16.

27. Ibid.

28. Schiavo I, 780 So. 2d at 179.

29. Petition for Writ of Certiorari, *Bush v. Schiavo*, No. 04–757, 2004 WL 2790640, at *4; available under the Timeline entry for March 23, 2005, at http://www.miami.edu/ethics/schiavo/schiavo_timeline.html.

30. Fla. Stat. ch. 744.309(1) (2004).

31. Petition for Writ of Certiorari, *Bush v. Schiavo*, No. 04–757, 2004 WL 2790640, at *16–17.

32. National Right to Life Committee Model Legislation, available at www. nrlc.org/euthanasia/ModelBillAnnouncement.html. See also Cerminara, K.L. Critical essay: Musings on the need to convince some people with disabilities that end-of-life decisionmaking advocates are not out to get them. *Loyola University Chicago Law Journal* 2006;37:343–384, 381–82 n. 231 (listing states considering such legislation).

33. Cantor, N.L. The relationship between autonomy-based rights and profoundly mentally disabled persons. *Annals of Health Law* 2004;13:37–80, 40.

34. Schiavo I, 780 So. 2d at 179.

35. Ibid.

36. *Cruzan*, 497 U.S. 261.

37. *In re Quinlan*, 355 A.2d 647, cert. denied sub nom *Garger v. New Jersey*, 429 U.S. 922 (1976).

38. Audio Tape: Fla. S. Spec. Sess. E at 2:57; Audio tape: Fla. H.R. Spec. Sess. E HB35-E at 1:00–1:04+.

39. "The Right to Die," ' 6.03[G] (table).

40. John Paul II, Address to the Participants in the International Congress on "Life- Sustaining Treatments and Vegetative State: Scientific Advances and Ethical Dilemmas," March 20, 2004, available at http://www.vatican. va/holy_father/john_paul_ii/speeches/ 2004/march/documents/ hf_jp-ii_spe_20040320_congress-fiamc_en.html.

41. "The Right to Die," ' 7.07[B] at text accompanying nn. 331, 332 (citing statutes).

42. Bernat, J.L., Gert, B., and Mogielnicki, R.P. Patient refusal of hydration and nutrition. An alternative to physician-assisted suicide or voluntary active euthanasia. *Archives of Internal Medicine* 1993;153:2723–2728, 2725–26.

43. Cerminara, "Critical Essay," 343–384, 381–82, n. 231 (listing states considering such legislation).

44. National Right to Life Committee Model Legislation, current version available at www.nrlc.org/euthanasia/ModelBillAnnouncement.html. The version of the act described in the text was the original version; the act since has been amended so that it provides only the first and second of these options.

5 ∷

The Continuing Assault on Personal
Autonomy in the Wake of the
Schiavo Case

Jon B. Eisenberg

∷ Core Values

Advance directives for health care have been slow to catch on with the American public since their inception in the late 1960s.[1] But that has changed in the wake of the *Schiavo* case. During the weeks surrounding Terri Schiavo's death in early 2005, hundreds of thousands of Americans flooded health care advocacy organizations and state bar associations with requests for advance directive forms.[2] Pre-*Schiavo* studies suggested that no more than 10 to 20 percent of Americans had given advance directives,[3] but by November 2005 a Pew Research Center study had that number surging to 29 percent.[4]

Health care professionals see this as good news. Some religious conservatives, however, are reacting with renewed and escalating assaults on advance directives and their bioethical underpinning: personal autonomy.

Some mainstream bioethicists have identified four central values underlying the traditions of Western medical practice:

- *Beneficence*—promoting the well-being of patients
- *Professional integrity*—deferring to the personal moral and religious beliefs of health care providers
- *Justice*—ensuring equal access to limited medical resources
- *Personal autonomy*—protecting patients' rights to retain control over their own bodies and to determine the nature of their medical care[5]

None of these four values trumps the others. But personal autonomy is given special weight,[6] and it is unique among the four in that it is rooted not just in the traditions of Western medical practice but also in American law. As early as 1891, in *Union Pacific Railway Co. v. Botsford*, the United States Supreme Court enunciated "the right of every individual to possession and control of his own person, free from all restraint or interference of others, unless by clear and unquestionable authority of law."[7] In the landmark 1990 case of *Cruzan v. Director, Missouri Dept. of Health*, the Supreme Court said that personal autonomy—which the Court called "bodily integrity"—includes the right to refuse medical treatment and is constitutionally guaranteed by the due process clause of the Fourteenth Amendment.[8]

The bioethical opposite of personal autonomy is *paternalism*—a values system that holds that health care decisions should be entrusted to doctors, family, community, and clergy rather than the individual alone. Paternalism still prevails in some countries but has long been disfavored in America.

All states now have legislation governing exercise of the constitutional right to refuse medical treatment, authorizing various types of advance directives for medical care and in some instances codifying "form advance directives" that will satisfy the requirements of state law. Additionally, federal law requires health care facilities to give patients information about their state-law rights to make advance directives.[9]

Legislation in Florida, where Terri Schiavo resided, is typical of state laws nationwide. The Florida State Legislature has declared that "every competent adult has the fundamental right of self-determination regarding decisions pertaining to his or her own health, including the right to choose or refuse medical treatment."[10] Florida Statutes prescribe standards for the exercise of this right on behalf of persons who have become incompetent, in order to "ensure that such right is not lost or diminished by virtue of later physical or mental incapacity."[11] If the patient has executed an advance directive that gives instructions concerning life-prolonging measures, those instructions are to be followed.[12] The Florida Statutes include a sample form living will, which may but need not be used.[13]

Of course, with some 70 percent of Americans still lacking advance directives, some sort of guidance is required for surrogate exercise of the right to refuse medical treatment where there is no advance directive. Accordingly, bioethicists have formulated three models for surrogate exercise of autonomy rights, with the goal of deciding how the patient would choose if he or she were able:

- *Advance directive*—If there is an advance directive giving instructions for future medical care, the surrogate follows the patient's instructions.
- *Substituted judgment*—If there is no advance directive or there is one but its instructions do not seem to cover the situation presented, and the patient previously had otherwise made his or her preferences and values known (for example, through conversations with the surrogate about end-of-life choices), the surrogate makes a decision based on the patient's subjective wishes, attempting to decide as the patient would have decided when competent.
- *Best interests*—If nothing is known about the patient's preferences and values, the surrogate makes a decision based on an objective assessment of the patient's best interests, attempting to decide as most people would choose under the circumstances.[14]

Here, there is a trump card: the patient's preferences and values, whether expressed in an advance directive or determined under the substituted judgment model. The best-interests model is one of last resort, to be invoked only when the others cannot be used.[15] As the advance-directive and substituted-judgment models are rooted in the central value of personal autonomy, that means personal autonomy trumps the values of beneficence, professional integrity, and justice in surrogate exercise of the right to refuse medical treatment.

State laws generally track these three bioethical models and the trumping nature of autonomy. Again, legislation in Florida is typical of state laws nationwide. Absent an advance directive giving instructions for future medical care, a Florida surrogate must make the health care decision that the surrogate "reasonably believes the patient would have made under the circumstances."[16] If there is no indication what the patient would have chosen, the surrogate "may consider the patient's best interest in deciding that proposed treatments are to be withheld or that treatments currently in effect are to be withdrawn."[17]

The denouement of the *Schiavo* case was a hard-fought triumph for American notions of personal autonomy. The trial judge, George Greer, acting as Terri Schiavo's surrogate under the substituted-judgment model, decided that her feeding tube should be removed because that was the decision *she* would have made. A group of Republican politicians, religious conservatives, disability-rights activists, and pro-life stalwarts strove mightily to overturn Judge Greer's decision—in state and federal appeals courts, in the Florida Legislature and governor's office, in the United States Congress, and in the White House. Those efforts—paternalistic at best and cynically opportunistic at worst—all failed. Autonomy prevailed.

And the result would have been the same under the best-interests model. Polls show that most Americans—up to 80 percent—would personally refuse life-sustaining treatment under Terri Schiavo's circumstances.[18]

:: The Assault on Advance Directives

During the *Schiavo* litigation, some religious conservatives reacted with an assault on personal autonomy in general and advance directives in particular. For example, in a series of articles posted on its website, Focus on the Family rejected the notion of choice in dying. One of the articles quotes the biblical injunction "that your body is a temple of the Holy Spirit who is in you, whom you have from God and that you are not your own" (1 Corinthians 6:19, 20).[19] Another article said the living will form of advance directive is to be "discouraged" as a "vague statement" that "[a]ttempts to predict your preferences in often complex medical situations that you cannot foresee by offering a narrow list of options that may be used to prohibit treatment you would want in a certain circumstance."[20]

The Christian Medical and Dental Associations argues: "Autonomy today typically means both that decisions critically affecting a patient's life should be made by the patient, and that whatever decision a patient makes is right simply by virtue of the fact that the patient has made it. A Christian perspective challenges both of these claims . . . . [W]hile affirming and protecting the individual, a biblical outlook also emphasizes the significance of community, which is rarely commended in an autonomy-based approach."[21]

Priests for Life, declaring that "[w]e do not have a 'right to die,'" said living wills "are unnecessary and dangerous for patients, doctors, and society" because, among other things, "the language used is too broad and can be open to a variety of interpretations." Living wills, said Priests for Life, are "not morally justified."[22]

In the months after Terri Schiavo's death, these attacks on personal autonomy and advance directives coalesced into a full-blown assault. At the vanguard was the President's Council on Bioethics, established by executive order of President George W. Bush.

In September 2005, the Council issued its book-length report, *Taking Care: Ethical Caregiving in Our Aging Society*. The report includes an entire chapter on "The Limited Wisdom of Advance Directives,"[23] which advocates a return to paternalism by making the bioethical central value of personal autonomy subservient to beneficence—a radical departure from mainstream bioethics.

Distinguishing between two types of advance directives—the "power of attorney for health care" or "proxy directive" appointing a surrogate decision-maker, and the "living will" or "instruction directive" specifying wanted or unwanted medical treatment (which are often combined in a single document)[24]—the report praises proxy directives but condemns living wills. The report says: "Living wills make autonomy and self-determination the primary values at a time of life when one is no longer autonomous or self-determining, and when what one needs is loyal and loving care."[25] In contrast, the report continues: "Proxy directives serve the wise and helpful purpose of putting one's trust explicitly in the hands of loved ones who rightly bear the burden of providing care and making decisions."[26] The report proposes a revisionist bioethical regime that is "focused not simply on discerning or executing an incompetent person's prior wishes but on providing the best care possible for the person now placed in our care."[27]

The report's assault on personal autonomy is unrelenting:

- "[T]here are serious reasons to doubt the wisdom of treating patient autonomy as the crucial guide for making end-of-life care decisions for patients who are, in fact, no longer autonomous but absolutely dependent on others for their care."[28]
- "A person's prior wishes and instructions surely count in any judgment about providing care. . . . But giving those wishes trumping power may force caregivers to forgo doing what is best for the person who is now entrusted to their care; as moral agents themselves, caregivers cannot simply do what they were told but must also try to do what is best."[29]
- "[H]owever much we understandably cling to our autonomy and dread our decline, dependency is very often part of the normal course of human life."[30]
- "Writing a living will requires facing up to the possibility of decline, debility, and death, but it does so by seeking to exert more self-mastery than may be possible at a time of life when accepting limits and trusting others are often the virtues most needed."[31]

- "Even when people are prepared to execute living wills, it is doubtful whether they have clear and definite ideas about the treatment they would want if and when they become incapacitated. There are, to begin with, simply too many possible future situations that the patient must try to imagine. . . ."[32]

The report concludes that a bioethical approach encouraging proxy directives but discouraging living wills "emphasizes less the importance of self-determination and correspondingly more the importance of solidarity and interdependence. . . . [T]he proxy directive is more in accord with our ideals of family and community life than is the instruction directive."[33]

∷ The Return of Paternalism

If there could be any doubt that the proposed approach is intended to give primacy to the best-interests model and make autonomy subservient to beneficence, it is dispelled by reference to a transcribed Council hearing on April 2, 2004, where the following exchange occurred between Council members Rebecca S. Dresser and Gilbert C. Meilaender:

> Meilaender: "[I]f you're prepared to override an advance directive on the grounds of current best interest, that means you really do want to give primary weight to the objective best interest standard, right?"
> Dresser: "Right."[34]

And so paternalism is back. Personal autonomy is but an illusion to which we foolishly cling. Our likely fate is dependence. We must place our trust in doctors, family, and community, not our own prescience, to decide what medical treatment is best for us in our dependency.

The Council's report echoes the voices of religious conservatives during the final months of the *Schiavo* litigation. Says Focus on the Family: "You are not your own,"[35] and the living will is a "vague statement" that "attempts to predict your preferences in often complex medical situations that you cannot foresee."[36] Says the Christian Medical and Dental Associations: "The best treatment refusal decisions are typically made together with one's physician, taking into account the well-being of family, friends, and others, and not merely oneself."[37] Sound familiar?

The report rightly points out that living wills are sometimes less than perfect: They can be misplaced or forgotten by the time they are needed,[38] and the instructions in form living wills can be vague and subject to conflicting interpretations.[39] Moreover, danger lurks whenever people attempt to write their own instructions with particularity, because of the near impossibility of foreseeing all the physical and mental misfortunes that might befall us. A detailed list of unacceptable circumstances might be treated as exclusive, meaning life will be sustained in whatever circumstances are not foreseen and listed.

But these are hardly reasons for abandoning living wills as some sort of failed experiment. As living wills continue to gain acceptance with an American public spurred on by the *Schiavo* case, their shortcomings will dissipate. The more routine advance directives become, the more routinely they will become a part of a patient's medical records so that there is less risk of their being misplaced or forgotten. The more people think and talk about end-of-life decision making in public dialogues and private conversations, the more care people will take in making their wishes known.

As for vagueness in form living wills, that is a problem only if one views them as attempts to foresee each and every possible future medical circumstance with particularity—which is not and should not be the goal of autonomy-based surrogate decision making. The goal is simply to decide how the patient would choose if he or she were able. That goal is most commonly achieved by knowing the patient's *preferences and values*, whether specified in an advance directive or made known to the surrogate in other ways such as conversations about end-of-life choices. It can be achieved as much by expressing one's general views on life and death as by attempting to list all the specific medical conditions that one would consider intolerable. If the expression is not specific enough to address a given medical condition and enable a decision under the "advance directive" model for surrogate exercise of autonomy rights, then it likely will shed enough light on the patient's preferences and values to enable a decision based on the autonomy-based "substituted judgment" model.

For example, the California Medical Association's form advance directive gives a choice between two instructions for a surrogate's guidance "if I am suffering from a terminal condition from which death is expected in a matter of months, or if I am suffering from an irreversible condition that renders me unable to make decisions for myself, and life-support treatments are needed to keep me alive":

- "I request that all treatments other than those needed to keep me comfortable be discontinued or withheld and my physician(s) allows me to die as gently as possible."
- "I want my life to be prolonged as long as possible within the limits of generally accepted health care standards."[40]

The choice is between two fundamentally different philosophies of life and death: "don't keep me alive on artificial life support if I am terminally ill or permanently incompetent," versus "do everything to keep me alive as long as possible." That ought to be enough to guide surrogates through most decisions, without the dangers of over-specificity. There will always be exceptional circumstances that fall into a gray area of ambiguity—which is why, absent adequate guidance from knowledge of the patient's preferences and values, bioethical principles and the law provide for an objective "best interests" decision.

∷ Resilience of Living Wills

How well living wills are working, however, is beside the point—which is that an ever-increasing number of Americans *want them.* According to the Pew Research Center, by the end of 2005 the number of Americans with living wills had risen to 29 percent, up from 12 percent in 1990.[41] That number is approaching the American Bar Foundation's estimate of 40 percent for Americans who have wills disposing of their estates,[42] and will continue to rise as attorneys increasingly make it routine practice to have clients execute advance directives at the same time they prepare a will. The 2005 percentages for living wills are even higher for older folks—49 percent in the 63-to-77-year age group, and 57 percent above age 77.[43] Personal autonomy remains an enduring value for most Americans, with 84 percent supporting "[l]aws that let patients decide about being kept alive through medical treatment."[44]

And people are talking more and more with their loved ones about end-of-life choices. According to the 2005 Pew Research Center study, nearly 70 percent of married persons have had conversations with their spouses about their wishes for end-of-life treatment, up from 51 percent in 1990.[45] Of adults with living parents, 57 percent have spoken with their mother, and 48 percent with their father, about the parent's wishes regarding end-of-life treatment.[46]

Living wills and dialogue about end-of-life decision making have become mainstream in an America that cherishes personal autonomy.

Religious conservative groups like Focus on the Family, the Christian Medical and Dental Associations, and Priests for Life—and the President's Council on Bioethics—have embraced an anti-autonomy dogma that represents the view of a small minority of Americans.

How can this assault on personal autonomy be repulsed? By continuing the drive to get Americans to make advance directives. In the wake of the *Schiavo* case, the execution of an advance directive has become a political act—an assertion of personal autonomy in the face of efforts to squelch that most basic of American rights. The more common advance directives become, the more difficult it will be for the likes of the President's Council on Bioethics to take them away from us.

NOTES TO CHAPTER 5

1. Attorney Luis Kutner proposed a "living will" in Kutner, L. Due Process of Euthanasia: The living will, a proposal," *Indiana Law Journal* 1969;44:539–534.
2. E.g., Schwartz, J., and Estrin, J. Many still seek one final say on ending life, *The New York Times*, June 17, 2005 (800,000 requests for "Five Wishes" advance directive from the nonprofit organization "Aging with Dignity" during March and early April of 2005); 17,000 download living wills from NY State Bar Assn. website, *Daily Record*, Rochester, N.Y., March 30, 2005.
3. California Law Revision Commission. *Recommendation: Health Care Decisions for Adults Without Decisionmaking Capacity*, California Law Revision Commission 1999;29:1–243 (publication 201), available at http://www.clrc.ca.gov/pub/Printed-Reports/Pub201.pdf; Pew Research Center for the People and the Press. More Americans Discussing—and Planning—End-of-Life Treatment: Strong Public Support for Right to Die, January 2006, available at http://people-press.org/reports/display.php3?ReportID=266.
4. Ibid.
5. Hastings Center Project on the Termination of Treatment and Care of the Dying. *Guidelines on the Termination of Life-Sustaining Treatment and the Care of the Dying*, Bloomington: Indiana University Press, 1987, pp. 6–8. The four central values identified by the members of the Hastings Center Project differ slightly from the four principles of respect for autonomy, beneficence, nonmaleficence, and justice identified by Tom L. Beauchamp and James F. Childress and developed through the several editions of their *Principles of Biomedical Ethics* (Oxford: Oxford University Press, 5th edition, 2001) in that the Hastings Center Project identifies "professional integrity" where Beauchamp and Childress identify "nonmaleficence" (not harming the patient). Nothing of great importance hangs on this difference; indeed, several important criticisms of and alternatives to the Beauchamp and Childress formulation have been proposed. The main point is the central role assigned to the concept of respect for personal autonomy.

6. Hastings Center, *Guidelines*, p. 8.
7. 141 U.S. 250, 251 (1891).
8. 497 U.S. 261, 269–270, 278–279 (1990).
9. Patient Self Determination Act, 42 U.S.C. § 1395cc(a)(1)(Q) & (f).
10. Florida Statutes, § 765.102(1).
11. Ibid.
12. Florida Statutes, § 765.302, § 765.304.
13. Florida Statutes, § 765.303.
14. Hastings Center, *Guidelines*, pp. 27–28.
15. Ibid., p. 28.
16. Florida Statutes, § 765.401(2).
17. Ibid.
18. E.g., Blanton, D. Majority would remove Schiavo's feeding tube. Fox News, June 18, 2004, available at http://www.foxnews.com/story/0,2933,101826,00.html (poll conducted by the Opinion Dynamics Corp. showed 74 percent of respondents would want a guardian to remove the tube); Langer, G. Poll: No role for government in Schiavo case—Federal intervention in Schiavo case prompts broad public disapproval, ABC News, March 21, 2005, available at http://abcnews.go.com/Politics/PollVault/story?id=599622&page=1 (poll conducted by TNS Intersearch found that 78 percent would not want a tube).
19. Earll, C.J. What the Bible says about the end of life. Citizen Link—Focus on Social Issues, February 27, 1998, available at http://www.citizenlink.org/FOSI/bioethics/A000001322.cfm.
20. Earll, C.J. Advance medical directives. Citizen Link—Focus on Social Issues, December 16, 2003, available at http://www.citizenlink.org/FOSI/bioethics/eoli/A000002155.cfm.
21. Christian Medical and Dental Associations. Advance directives, Statement of April 29, 1994, available at http://www.cmda.org.
22. Pavone, F.A. Brief reflections on euthanasia, No date, available at
23. http://www.priestsforlife.org/euthanasia/euthrefl.html.
24. President's Council on Bioethics. *Taking Care: Ethical Caregiving in Our Aging Society.* Washington: President's Council on Bioethics, 2005, pp. 53–93.
25. Ibid., pp. 57–58.
26. Ibid., p. 55.
27. Ibid.
28. Ibid., p. 56.
29. Ibid., p. 80.
30. Ibid., p. 84.
31. Ibid., p. 88.
32. Ibid.
33. Ibid., p. 73.
34. Ibid., p. 89.
35. Transcript of President's Commission on Bioethics, Session 6: Bioethical Issues of Aging II: The Wisdom of Advance Directives, April 2, 2004, available at http://bioethics.gov/transcripts/april04/april2full.html.

36. Earll. "What the Bible says."
37. Earll. "Advance medical directives."
38. Christian Medical and Dental Associations. "Advance directives."
39. President's Council on Bioethics. *Taking Care.* p. 75.
40. Ibid., pp. 73–75.
41. California Medical Association. Introduction to Advance Health Care Directives, available at http://www.cmanet.org/member/upload/AdvDirSample2005.pdf.
42. Pew Research Center. "End-of Life-Treatment."
43. McMillan, A.F. People don't like to plan for their death, but avoiding it is a financial mistake. CNN Money, August 31, 1999, available at http://money.cnn.com/1999/08/31/life/q_will/.
44. Pew Research Center. "End-of Life-Treatment."
45. Ibid.
46. Ibid.
47. Ibid.

6 ::

A Common Uniqueness: Medical Facts in the Schiavo Case

Ronald E. Cranford

:: Introduction

The controversial issues in the Terri Schiavo case were extremely common, and extraordinarily unique.

Every day in the United States, tubes that provide artificial nutrition and hydration (ANH) are withdrawn from patients in a permanent vegetative state (PVS). No one knows the exact number, but it is a common occurrence.

And every day in the United States, some families are completely unable to accept the reality of the diagnosis of a PVS. They will never to be able to accept the neurological facts that their loved one is unconscious and has no chance of recovery—just like Mary and Robert Schindler, the parents of Terri Schiavo.

Recent advances in medical treatment, especially cardiopulmonary resuscitation, have resulted in a marked increase in the frequency of PVS patients in contemporary society. Major differences among members of the immediate family about the appropriateness of further treatment are not uncommon. In this regard, mothers, because of the special bond between mothers and their children, seem to be the ones who have the most difficulty accepting the certainty of the outcome and the ones most strongly opposed to withdrawing treatment, even in the face of an overwhelmingly poor prognosis.

So the conflicts in the Schiavo case will be faced again and again in the future: A young person is in a PVS secondary to a tragic circumstance;

the spouse finally accepts the reality; but the parents or other family members cannot bring themselves to acknowledge the neurological facts and refuse to make any considerations about stopping treatment. Yet in my personal and professional experience—as a consulting neurology expert in landmark right-to-die cases over three decades—I have never observed anything remotely approaching the extraordinary and bizarre developments in Schiavo, and I hope I never will again. With respect to the neurological facts alone, the primary subject of this chapter, the Schiavo case was distinct from all other landmark right-to-die cases because of the following features:

1. The overwhelming and indisputable evidence of the neurological condition, including eventually the ultimate confirmatory findings in the autopsy
2. The longest and most comprehensive evidentiary hearing on the neurological facts
3. In the face of these facts, the remarkable and medically unsupported testimony by two experts stating in court that the patient was definitely not in a PVS and could respond to various treatments
4. Unequivocal and definitive opinions by the presiding trial court judge on the neurological facts, with a detailed review of the medical evidence and concurrence by the appellate court justices; and the most comprehensively litigated case (on the neurological facts alone, as well as other issues) in the history of the right-to-die movement
5. The effective use of videotapes by medical experts in the courtroom to educate the judge on aspects of the PVS; and the effective use of videotapes by others to mislead the public, the media, and politicians about Ms. Schiavo's condition
6. The unprecedented submission of a large number of erroneous affidavits to the court
7. The propaganda campaign by special interest groups to mislead the public about the process of terminal dehydration by calling it "starvation"
8. The mistaken diagnoses and denial of reality in the halls of Congress and elsewhere
9. The attempted use of a neurologist from a credible medical organization to deceive the court and public in the last days of Ms. Schiavo's life

10. The most comprehensive, accurate, and useful autopsy and medical examiner's report in any landmark right-to-die case
11. The continued denial of reality of the neurological facts by the family, the medical experts representing the Schindlers, and other advocates

These 11 features need to be described in greater detail.

:: The Neurological Evidence

From the very beginning of the case, at least when husband Michael Schiavo first attempted to withdraw the feeding tube in 1998, the heart of the Schindlers' and their representatives' (hereafter the "opponents") objections to this action rested on two factual issues: that Ms. Schiavo was not in a PVS, as asserted by her husband; and that Mr. Schiavo was not a fit guardian for his wife. Both of these factual assertions were eventually proved to be false.

The facts of Ms. Schiavo's neurological condition were extensively reviewed by Florida courts in at least four judicial decisions, and in professional journals by me and others.[1] Indeed, many of the facts are well known. On the early morning of February 25, 1990, Ms. Schiavo was found unconscious by her husband in their home. When paramedics arrived, they found her unresponsive and in ventricular fibrillation. She was subsequently defibrillated seven times with eventual restoration of normal heartbeat and blood pressure. She was in a coma for a few weeks, followed by opening of the eyes but no apparent conscious interactions with family. Over the next 12 years, until the evidentiary hearing by Judge George Greer in October 2002, four separate neurologists consulting on her case diagnosed PVS secondary to hypoxic-ischemic encephalopathy from the cardiac arrest. During those 12 years there was never any dispute among Ms. Schiavo's four consulting neurologists or her attending physicians about her neurological condition.

I was first alerted to the case in early 2001 by one of Ms. Schiavo's neurologists, Dr. James Barnhill. He briefly reviewed the case with me and asked if I would be willing to become involved. In the spring of 2002, George Felos, the lawyer representing Michael Schiavo, called me and asked if I would be willing to review the medical records and tests results, examine Ms. Schiavo, and then testify at an evidentiary hearing later in the year. He asked about my fees, and I told him that I usually served on a *pro bono* basis (except, hopefully, reimbursement for expenses) for these types of cases.

I examined Ms. Schiavo on July 20, 2002, in the presence of her husband, her parents, and Mr. Felos. My examination lasted 42 minutes. The parents were unable to stay for the entire examination. Ms. Schiavo's eyes were open throughout most of the examination, but at no time was there any visual pursuit or visual fixation. The eyes moved about randomly. At the beginning of the examination, while the parents were still present, I asked Ms. Schiavo's mother if her daughter could respond to commands in any consistent way, and she said no. The patient's head was turned to the right during most of the examination. She did have a consistent startle response to loud noises, such as hand clapping. Severe contractures were present in all four extremities. Stimulation by pinching a fold of skin under the arms produced decorticate posturing in the arms but no movement of the legs and no facial grimacing. There was no response to visual threat. She had a definite positive sucking reflex, increased jaw jerk, and an abnormal glabellar sign (or Myerson's sign, a primitive reflex in which patients cannot stop blinking when tapped repeatedly on the glabella, or the space between the eyebrows).

Only one minor clinical feature during my examination raised any question about the diagnosis of PVS. Throughout my entire examination, and during the hours of videotapes by all the other physicians, as well as the years of observation by Ms. Schiavo's treating doctors, there has never been any evidence of sustained (consistent and reproducible) visual pursuit, or visual tracking, usually the cardinal feature that distinguishes PVS from other, higher levels of consciousness, such as the minimally conscious state.[2] However, when I was testing for visual tracking with a brightly colored balloon in different fields of gaze, it appeared for about 15 seconds that Ms. Schiavo was following the balloon with her eyes both up and down and less so to the right and left. This brief period of apparent tracking did not in any way constitute sustained visual pursuit. It could have been a random response of the eyes, a brain stem auditory orienting response (following my voice instead of the balloon), or possibly a primitive visual orienting reflex, sometimes seen in PVS patients, and mediated via subcortical pathways in the brain stem and thalamus. Attempts to reproduce these same eye movements with the balloon later in my examination were unsuccessful. But these few seconds, taken out of context—namely, everything else we know about the diagnosis, including the opinions of credible physicians over 12 years and the clear documentation of severe, irreversible brain damage—became a powerful piece of propaganda for political conservatives. Even the videotapes released by the Schindler family and later used as a basis for health care professionals submitting affidavits do not show any sustained visual pursuit. But this has been a major strategy of those conservatives: to take some small and insignificant issue, wrench it out of context, and make it into a major point of contention.

The most recent CT scans, done in 1996 and 2002, showed incredibly severe atrophy of the cerebral hemispheres and other parts of the brain, which is exactly what a neurologist would expect from a patient in a PVS for 12 years. The two electroencephalograms done in 2002 showed no electrical activity (that is, the EEGs were flat), although the background activity was obscured to some extent by artifact. EEGs in PVS cases usually demonstrate very abnormal slowing but are very rarely flat, as in Ms. Schiavo's case. The CT scans were important because they demonstrated to the highest degree of medical certainty that Ms. Schiavo's condition was irreversible, and that no treatment of any kind would ever benefit her. The EEGs were important because they demonstrated objectively that she was not conscious, and just strongly confirmed the clinical diagnosis of PVS. None of the previous landmark cases that I am familiar with had demonstrated a flat EEG.

After my clinical examination and review of her medical records, EEGs, and CT scans, there was no doubt whatsoever that Ms. Schiavo fit all the criteria for the PVS. The findings on my examination were all consistent with a classic PVS and consistent with the clinical diagnosis that she had carried for 12 years.

I have always maintained that the vast majority of Americans would not want to be kept alive in a PVS. An ABC News poll conducted shortly before Ms. Schiavo's death asked, "If you were in this condition, would you want to be kept alive, or not?" Responses: 87% said they would not want continued treatment; 8% said they would.

∷ A Comprehensive Evidentiary Hearing

At the initial hearing in the case in 2000, Ms. Schiavo's primary attending physician and consulting neurologist testified that she was in a PVS. There was no medical testimony to the contrary at these initial court hearings, as Ms. Schiavo had carried an undisputed diagnosis of PVS for 10 years.

In Judge Greer's order of February 2000, he ruled that Terri Schiavo's previous oral declarations, including "I don't want to be kept alive on a machine," were "reliable" and "credible" and rose to "the level of clear and convincing evidence," consistent with the substituted judgment standard adopted by the Florida Supreme Court in two separate decisions, *John F Kennedy Memorial Hospital v Bludworth* in 1984 and *Browning* in 1990. Additionally, Judge Greer found that, "beyond all doubt," based on "overwhelming credible evidence" from the testimony of Dr. Vincent Gambone, Ms. Schiavo's treating physician, and Dr. Barnhill, one of the consulting neurologists, she was in a persistent vegetative state as defined by Florida Statue 765.101.[3]

When the case was on appeal to Florida's Second District Court of Appeals, the higher court took note of several affidavits submitted to the court, including one by Dr. Fred Webber, an osteopathic physician in Clearwater, Florida, to the effect that Ms. Schiavo was not in a PVS and had the potential to respond to treatment. Even though the appellate court viewed this affidavit with some skepticism, the justices decided to order a full-scale evidentiary hearing exclusively on the neurological condition of the patient. This hearing required that at least six physicians testify about that neurological condition: Ms. Schiavo's primary attending physician, two experts selected by Michael Schiavo, two selected by the Schindler family, and one other expert either agreed to by both sides, or, in case the two sides could not agree, an expert selected by the judge. The doctors would then each be given one full day in court to give their opinions and be subjected to direct and cross examination by the opposing parties.[4]

The hearing took place over six days in October 2002 and Ms. Schiavo's neurological condition was addressed in testimony by the six physicians: Victor Gambone, the primary attending physician caring for her for many years; William Maxfield, a radiologist, and William M. Hammesfahr, a neurologist, representing the Schindler family; Melvin Greer and myself, neurologists, representing Michael Schiavo; and the expert appointed by the court, Peter Bambakidis, from Cleveland, Ohio. Each doctor was given one full day in court for his testimony and opinions, allowing plenty of time for direct and cross examination by the attorneys representing Michael Schiavo and Mary and Robert Schindler.

At this evidentiary hearing the videotapes were played, and the 1996 and 2002 CT scans were shown and extensively discussed with the court. Some experts emphasized at trial that extensive neurological changes indicated permanent damage to the brain and confirmed beyond any doubt the irreversibility of Ms. Schiavo's brain damage; they demonstrated persuasively that she never was a candidate for any form of therapy, let alone the untested, unapproved, and therefore completely inappropriate treatments of hyperbaric oxygen and vasodilator therapy advocated by Drs. Maxfield and Hammesfahr respectively.

:: Flawed Expert Testimony

At the evidentiary hearing the two physicians representing the Schindler family testified that Ms. Schiavo was not in a PVS and could respond to treatment. One of them, Dr. Maxfield, the radiologist, was not qualified to do a *neurological* examination and did not in fact perform such an examination, as clearly seen in his videotape. The other, Dr. Hammesfahr, a neurologist, has said he observed Terri Schiavo over a period of 10 hours, mistakenly implying that the duration of the examination should add to its credibility. His examination was in fact not a comprehensive neurological examination, but more a prolonged "conversation with Terri" about how well she was doing and how much she was cooperating with him and "interacting" with her parents.

One of the case's major recurrent questions is this: If the opponents were so sure that Ms. Schiavo was not PVS, why didn't they retain believable, highly qualified experts to examine her and present a credible impression for the courts? No one can answer this question except those who retained Drs. Maxfield and Hammesfahr, but I strongly suspect that the medical records had already been reviewed by competent neurologists prior to the evidentiary hearing, who undoubtedly told the opponents that Ms. Schiavo was in fact in a PVS. So, as ineffective as they were, Drs. Hammesfahr and Maxfield were the best available. These two doctors had advocated hyperbaric oxygen therapy and vasodilator therapy for other patients with severe brain damage, both treatments of no value whatsoever in such situations. Their attempts to convince the judge of the worthiness of these treatments were completely dismissed by the court.

Judge Greer did not have any difficulty recognizing the invalidity of these experts' examinations, recommendations for treatment, and conclusions.[5] Judge Greer wrote in November 2002 (in an order that the feeding tube be removed):

> It is clear that this [vasodilation] therapy is not recognized in the medical community. Dr. Hammesfahr operates his clinic on a cash

basis in advance which made the discussion regarding Medicare eligibility quite irrelevant. A lot of the time also was spent regarding his nominations for a Nobel Prize. While he certainly is a self-promoter and should have had for the court's review a copy of the letter from the Nobel committee in Stockholm, Sweden, the truth of the matter is that he is probably the only person involved in these proceedings who had a United States congressman recommend him for such an award. Whether the committee "accepted" the nomination, "received" the nomination or whatever, it is not that significant. What is significant, however, and what undermines his creditability is that he did not present to this court any evidence other than his generalized statements as to the efficacy of his therapy on brain damaged individuals like Terry [sic] Schiavo. He testified that he has treated about 50 patients in the same or worse condition than Terry Schiavo since 1994 but he offered no names, no case studies, no videos and no tests results to support his claim that he had success in all but one of them. *If his therapy is as effective as he would lead this court to believe, it is inconceivable that he would not produce clinical results of these patients he has treated. And surely the medical literature would be replete with this new, now patented, procedure.* Yet, he has only published one article and that was in 1995 involving some 63 patients, 60% of whom were suffering from whiplash. None of these patients were in a persistent vegetative state and all were conversant. Even he acknowledges that he is aware of no article or study that shows vasodilatation therapy to be an effective treatment for persistent vegetative state patients. The court can only assume that such substantiations are not available, not just catalogued in such a way that they cannot be readily identified as he testified.[6]

:: Unequivocal Court Rulings

Judge Greer was most impressed with the testimony of Dr. Bambakidis, the court-appointed expert, and least impressed with the testimony of Drs. Maxfield and Hammesfahr. He wrote in conclusion that:

> The court finds that the credible evidence overwhelmingly supports the view that Terry [sic] Schiavo remains in a vegetative state. . . . It is clear from the evidence that these therapies [hyperbaric oxygen and vasodilatation] are experimental insofar as the medical community is concerned with regard to patients like Terry Schiavo *which is borne out by the total absence of supporting case studies or medical literature. . . . The other doctors, by contrast, all testified there was no treatment available to improve her quality of life.* They were also able to credibly testify that neither hyperbaric therapy nor vasodilatation therapy was an effective treatment for this sort of injury.[7]

Even though the Second District Court of Appeals could have affirmed the trial court opinion on procedural grounds (ensuring that the guidelines for the evidentiary hearing were properly executed) and gone no further, the court did go further and ruled on the factual issues as well. "Despite our decision that the appropriate standard of review is abuse of discretion [by Judge Greer], this court has closely examined all of the evidence in this record. We have repeatedly examined the videotapes, not merely watching short segments but carefully observing the tapes in their entirety. We have examined the brain scans with the eyes of educated laypersons and considered the explanations provided by the doctors in transcripts. We have concluded that, if we were called upon to review the guardianship's decision de novo, we would still affirm it."[8]

One reason the appellate court ordered a detailed evidentiary hearing on the medical facts of the case was that it received sworn affidavits by the Schindler family's doctors and other health care professionals stating that new treatments might improve Ms. Schiavo's level of functioning. As the court noted, " . . . Although we have expressed some lay skepticism about the new affidavits, the Schindlers now have presented some evidence, in the form of the affidavit of Dr. [Fred] Webber, of such a potential new treatment." Later, the court "anticipated but did not require that Dr. Webber, who had claimed in his affidavit that he might be able to restore Mrs. Schiavo's speech and some of her cognitive functioning, would testify for the parents and provide scientific support for his claim. However, Dr. Webber, who was so critical in this court's decision to remand the case, made no further appearance in these proceedings."[9]

Why did the three judges on the court of appeals bend over backwards these many years to listen carefully to the concerns of the Schindlers, including ordering a full-scale evidentiary hearing on Ms. Schiavo's medical condition after all the other legal issues had been fully litigated, and after the trial court judge had ruled in February 2000 that Terri Schiavo was in a PVS "beyond all doubt?" Beside the obvious and to some extent understandable motivation of judges to avoid error (especially on medical diagnosis), their natural tendency to err on the side of life (rather than erring on the side of privacy), and their appropriate concern about due process in cases of a highly controversial nature, a partial answer to this question has been supplied directly by the judges themselves. By revealing a human side of their decision-making process (something many judges are not usually willing to admit), they explicitly reflect their great sympathy and empathy toward the parents of Terri Schiavo:

> "The judges on this panel are called upon to make a collective, objective decision concerning a question of law. Each of us, however, has our own family, our own loved ones, our own children. From our review of the videotapes of Mrs. Schiavo, despite the irrefutable evidence that her cerebral cortex has sustained the most severe of irreparable injuries, we understand why a parent who has raised and nurtured a child since conception would hold out hope that some level of cognitive function remained. If Mrs. Schiavo were our own daughter, we could not but hold to such faith."[10]

In other words, the judges, while sympathetic to the feelings and concerns of the Schindlers, nevertheless based their decisions on the facts and the law.

So the view that Terri Schiavo was not in a PVS was pure propaganda on the part of vocal opponents, and wishful thinking in the minds of the Schindler family—a loving, caring family that just could not accept (and apparently never will) the reality of the bleak prognosis.

:: The Use of Videotapes to Educate—and Deceive

When I realized how elaborate the evidentiary hearing would be, I told attorney George Felos that I would request my examination be videotaped and that I hoped the other physicians would have their examinations videotaped as well. Unlike all previous right-to-die cases in which I have had a role, this was the first time a videotape would be made and then played in court in order for a judge to see the examination and verify the findings of the expert witness. I had no idea, at that time, how important these videotapes would be in this case. However, based on my previous courtroom experience, I felt a videotape would add credibility to my examination and enable me to show the trial court judge my findings and to explain the significance of these findings. I noted there was considerable reticence on the part of the doctors selected by the Schindler family to make a videotape of their examination, but eventually they did agree to this. Dr. Bambakidis, the expert appointed by the court, agreed to a videotape, but the other expert selected by Michael Schiavo, Melvin Greer, a previous president of the American Academy of Neurology, declined, as did the primary treating physician.

With respect to the opinions of Dr. Hammesfahr and the correlation of his findings with the videotape of his examination, Judge Greer noted: "Dr. Hammesfahr testified . . . he gave 105 commands . . . Mrs. Schindler gave an additional 6 commands . . . he asked her 61 questions and Mrs. Schindler, at his direction, asked her an additional 11 questions [for a total of 183 attempts]. The court saw few actions that could be considered responsive to either these commands or those questions. While Dr. Hammesfahr testified that she squeezed his finger on command, the video would not appear to support that and his reaction on the video likewise would not appear to support that testimony."[11]

The videotapes of the neurological examinations proved to be extremely successful in demonstrating PVS in the courtroom, far beyond my expectations. The tapes of the credible medical experts gave the judge an opportunity to see firsthand the clinical findings and allowed the experts to explain these findings to the court. And the videotapes of the experts retained by the Schindler family demonstrated to the judge the complete lack of credibility of their examinations and their opinions.

In preparation for the evidentiary hearing of October 2002, four hours of videotape of interactions were made between the doctors examining Ms. Schiavo and interactions among Ms. Schiavo, her family, and the doctors. These videotapes in turn were shown at the evidentiary hearing. As above, the tapes were crucial in convincing Judge Greer and the appellate court justices that Ms. Schiavo was indeed in a PVS. Judge Greer then ordered all parties not to "disseminate" these tapes to the public "in any way." However, the Schindlers and their representatives edited excerpts of these four hours down to six separate segments lasting a total of 4 minutes and 28 seconds. These excerpts were then released in a campaign to lead the public to believe that Ms. Schiavo was not in a PVS, and to induce various health care professionals into filing affidavits with erroneous opinions about her neurological condition. This propaganda campaign using the videotapes was enormously successful in misleading the American people, the vast majority of whom had never seen a PVS patient before.

:: The Affidavit Blizzard

As the *Schiavo* case wound through the courts, and media attention markedly increased, the political conservatives who attached themselves to the case resorted to an increasing number of desperate measures to defend their position on the two fundamental factual issues of the case: First, that Ms. Schiavo was not in a PVS and was capable of improving with appropriate treatment, and, second, that Michael Schiavo was not the appropriate surrogate for his wife.

One of the coordinated strategies was the submission to the courts of affidavits signed by various health care professionals (many with strong pro-life biases) that alleged Ms. Schiavo was not in a PVS and that her condition could be improved with treatment. These affidavits resulted from a systemic, nationwide effort to enlist the aid of physicians to dispute the clinical diagnosis of PVS. Much of this effort was coordinated through Dr. Thomas Zabeiga, a neurologist in Joliet, Illinois, and Batza & Associates, an investigation and litigation support business in Valencia, California, which was, in turn, was working for the Florida law firm of David Gibbs, the Schindlers' attorney. All told, Florida's judicial system received 33 affidavits. Many of these opinions were based on these brief videotapes released by the Schindler family and their supporters in direct violation of the court's order.

No physician, neurologist, or other health care professional would normally submit an affidavit to a court based on such findings as those in a brief videotape. Nor would any health care professional normally ever submit a written report to the court without a review of the relevant medical records and laboratory studies and a complete examination of the patient. But this is exactly what Dr. William Cheshire did late in the course of events when the conservatives became frantic to do anything they could to stop the inevitable flow of legal events leading to Ms. Schiavo's death.

These affidavits were not expressions of medical opinion as much as acts of political advocacy. Among other assertions, their signers claimed that the fact that Ms. Schiavo could handle her own oral secretions was indicative of her being outside the vegetative state. That was medically false: Vegetative patients are prone to pneumonia and other respiratory complications, a major cause of death, but they can usually handle daily oral secretions by the intact involuntary swallowing reflex. The affiants also stressed that Ms. Schiavo showed evidence of visual pursuit and fixation, but this was merely a figment of their imagination, or, more properly, an illusion and incorrect assertion based on their strong philosophical feelings and their misunderstanding of the essential features of a PVS diagnosis. Many argued forcefully that Ms. Schiavo was still a candidate for treatment. As the autopsy made clear when its results were released in June 2005, the opinions contained in the affidavits were completely false.

:: The Propaganda Campaign: Dehydration as "Starvation"

The withdrawal of artificial hydration and nutrition tubes from severely brain-damaged patients is not uncommon in contemporary medicine. I have been directly involved in the withdrawal of feeding tubes from PVS patients 25 to 50 times since the late 1970s. During the Paul Brophy case in Massachusetts in the 1980s, the first national right-to-die case involving removing hydration and nutrition from a PVS patient, political conservatives gave a long list of clinical features that occur during the process, which they characterized as "starvation." Since the mid-1980s, these partisans have continued to characterize the process of terminal dehydration as an agonizing process of starvation. This is a total distortion of the clinical reality.[12]

Since Brophy died in 1986, conservatives have chanted the same mantra over and over again, without major changes, despite all the evidence to the contrary—including considerable clinical experience and an extensive professional literature—that death after removal of the tube results in dehydration, not starvation. Of course, "starvation" sounds so much worse. Former U.S. House majority Leader, Tom DeLay, got into the act, decrying " . . . That Americans would be so barbaric as to pull a feeding tube out of a person that is lucid and starve them to death in two weeks."[13]

In response to a Schiavo-inspired bill pending in the Florida Legislature (HB701 "Starvation and Dehydration of Persons with Disabilities Prevention Act,"), Florida's leading bioethicists offered the following opinion on March 10, 2005:

> It is therefore essential to put in bold face the fact that terms like "starvation," as used in the title of HB701, are inaccurate, confusing and emotion-laden. Everyone rightly agrees that "starving someone to death" is abhorrent. But to suggest that the withdrawal or withholding of medically supplied artificial hydration and nutrition constitutes such a thing is medically false, morally mistaken and socially misleading. It would be a tragedy for the people of Florida if our Legislature were to make this error.[14]

The actual process of terminal dehydration occurs within a period of 10 to 14 days. For the first 7 to 10 days, no noticeable changes are seen. In the last 4 to 6 days significant changes result from the marked dehydration. There is a generalized loss of weight, most noticeably in the face, with sunken eyes and hollow cheeks, along with extreme dryness in the mucous membranes of the eyes and mouth. In the last few days of life, the distal extremities become cold and mottled, indicating an impending failure of the circulatory system and hypotension. In the last few hours the patient may slip into a coma, with respirations becoming increasingly slowed and shallower, and finally stopping.

Nancy Cruzan died of terminal dehydration in 11 days, 11.5 hours, and Christine Busalacchi in 11 days, 14 hours.[15] Terri Schiavo died of the same process in 12 days, 19 hours, and 45 minutes. She did not die of starvation. In the medical examiner's report discussed in the next section, the immediate cause of death was clear-cut. "She died of marked dehydration," wrote Dr. Jon Thogmartin, the medical examiner for Florida's Pinellas and Pasco counties, noting that the official cause of death would be listed as "complications of anoxic encephalopathy." At a news conference held on the day of the release of the report, the following interchange occurred:

> Reporter: "In layman's terms, did Terri Schiavo starve to death?"
> Thogmartin: "No."

Yet well after Ms. Schiavo's death, the Schindler family was still insisting that she was starved and dehydrated to death, writing to the Terri Schindler Schiavo Foundation website (Terrisfight.org), "Watching someone being starved and dehydrated to death, let alone your own daughter, is something so cruel that it can never be forgotten. . . . No, we will never forget the agonizing starvation death Terri suffered. Nor will we ever rest until each and every one of the perpetrators who orchestrated Terri's death is brought to justice for their crime against humanity."[16]

:: Mistaken Diagnoses

Many politicians, including the physician-politicians in Congress, made fools of themselves in offering clinical diagnoses by relying on brief videotapes released by the Schindler family, on descriptions of her condition by members of the Schindler family, and on the observations and opinions of Dr. Hammesfahr, whose testimony in the evidentiary hearing of 2002 was discredited by the presiding judge. At the same time, these politicians ignored or dismissed the clinical diagnosis of Ms. Schiavo's condition by four consulting neurologists directly involved in her care, by the trial testimony of the three neurologists whom the trial court judge found very credible (including the independent medical expert appointed by the judge himself), and the conclusion reached by the special guardian *ad litem*, Prof. Jay Wolfson, appointed to evaluate her condition.[17] These politicians also ignored the opinion of the trial court judge and the three-judge appeals court in Florida, which, after reviewing all of the medical evidence presented, found beyond any doubt that Ms. Schiavo had been in a "persistent" (permanent) vegetative state for 12 years.

Of all the health care professionals and physician-politicians who never examined Ms. Schiavo and never reviewed her medical records, the expert medical testimony, or the confirmatory laboratory studies, U.S. Rep. Dave Weldon, from Melbourne, Florida, self-described as a "hard-core Conservative," takes the prize for a complete denial of reality:

- "I practiced medicine for 15 years prior to my election to the House of Representatives. I still see patients once a month, and I was involved in numerous cases involving situations like this. . . . . Terry [sic] has been described in the press as being in a vegetative state, and I believe she is not, absolutely that she is not. . . ."[18]
- " . . . I am certain if doctors put an EEG on her, we would see extensive brain waves indicating activity in the visual cortex and in the speech centers . . ."[19]
- "It is not a person in the vegetative state. She has an active EEG. . . ."[20]
- "This is unprecedented for a judge to order the withdrawal of food and water from somebody. It has never been done before to my knowledge. . . . ."[21]

Now let's listen to Senator Bill Frist, at the time the Senate majority leader and, previously, a cardiac transplant surgeon:

Persistent vegetative state, which is what the court has ruled, I say I question it, and I question it based on a review of the video footage which I spent an hour or so looking at last night in my office here at the Capitol. And that footage, to me, depicted something very different than persistent vegetative state . . . there is no question in the video that she actually looks up . . . she certainly seems to respond to visual stimuli that the neurologist puts forth. . . . if you are going to allow somebody to die, starve them to death, I would think you would want to complete a neurological exam.[22]

Later, after the results of the autopsy were released, and the diagnosis of PVS was confirmed beyond any doubt, Senator Frist denied he questioned an attending physician's diagnosis. Frist's denial has led Jon Eisenberg to comment, "How stupid or forgetful does Frist think the American people are?"[23]

In 2004, vice presidential candidate Senator John Edwards said that Christopher Reeve "was a powerful voice for the need to do stem cell research and change the lives of people like him . . ." In October of that year, Senator Frist responded to Edwards' comments. "I find it opportunistic to use the death of someone like Christopher Reeve—I think it is shameful—in order to mislead the American people," Frist said. "We should be offering people hope, but neither physician, scientists, public servants or trial lawyers like John Edwards should be offering hype. . . . It is cruel to people who have disabilities and chronic diseases, and, on top of that, it's dishonest. It's giving false hope to people, and I can tell you as a physician who's treated scores of thousands of patients that you don't give them false hope."[24] Perhaps Senator Frist should take his own advice after treating "scores of thousands of patients."

Listen also to former U.S. House Majority Leader Tom DeLay: "Terri Schiavo is not brain-dead; she talks and she laughs, and she expresses happiness and discomfort. Terri Schiavo is not on life support."[25]

To be sure, denial of medical facts for political reasons was at least as interesting among nonphysicians. Barbara Weller, one of the lawyers representing the Schindlers, visited Ms. Schiavo on March 18, 2005. In a last-minute affidavit filed as part of broad attempt to restore Ms. Schiavo's artificial hydration and nutrition, Ms. Weller wrote, "I took her arms in both of my hands . . . I begged her to try very hard to say. 'I want to live.' To my enormous shock and surprise, Terri's eyes opened wide, she looked me square in the face, and with a look of great concentration, she said, 'Ahhhhhhh.' Then, seeming to summon up all the strength she had, she virtually screamed 'Waaaaaaaa.' . . . I promised Terri I would tell the world that she had tried to say 'I want to live.'"[26]

Even after the bedside observations of Barbara Weller about Ms. Schiavo's last-minute "pleas" that she wanted to live, the conservatives shifted to yet another desperate measure: They argued that her neurological condition had not been fully evaluated. They strongly urged that she undergo evaluation with newer, more sophisticated functional neuroimaging studies, specifically an fMRI and PET scans. But Judge Greer refused these motions, as he should have. Why weren't an fMRI and PET scan done in Ms. Schiavo's last days? There are several compelling reasons. First and foremost, these tests simply weren't medically indicated. By then, after the most extensively litigated case in the history of the right-to-die movement on the medical facts alone, as well as on the major legal issues, there was no doubt whatsoever in the minds of the treating physicians, the credible medical experts, and all the judges who had directly reviewed the medical evidence, that she had been in a PVS for 15 years. Second, it was patently obvious to anyone closely involved in the case, including Judge Greer, that the request for further studies was but one of a whole series of last-minute motions made by the Schindlers to prevent Ms. Schiavo's death. This point is convincingly demonstrated by the fact that the Schindlers continue to refuse to accept the definitive results of the autopsy. Third, an fMRI was contraindicated because of the implanted neural stimulator in Ms. Schiavo's brain, left over from an unsuccessful treatment attempt in 1990. As part of the final autopsy report, a letter from Dr. Stephen J. Nelson, a consulting neuropathologist who participated in the autopsy, notes that " . . . the U.S. Food and Drug Administration (FDA) issued an advisory to healthcare professionals that serious injury or death can occur when patients with implanted neurological stimulators—such as the decedent's implanted thalamic stimulator— undergo MRI (magnetic resonance imaging) procedures."[27] Fourth, there is simply not enough experience with these new functional studies as a definitive means to distinguish PVS or minimally conscious state to warrant their use in this case.

:: 11th-Hour Expert

Toward the end, when Ms. Schiavo was in the process of dying from terminal dehydration, the Schindlers and their representatives made an extraordinary, unprecedented series of last-minute legal and other maneuvers. One of these included enlisting the assistance of a neurologist who had "observed" Ms. Schiavo at her beside for 45 minutes and then submitted a detailed report to the court on her condition on March 23, 2005, five days after the feeding tube had been removed.

Dr. William Cheshire, a neurologist from the Mayo Clinic in Jacksonville, Florida, believed that "within a reasonable degree of medical certainty, there is a greater likelihood that Terri is in a minimally conscious state rather than a persistent vegetative state."[28] Dr. Cheshire never reviewed the EEGs, CT scans, or the testimony of medical experts at the evidentiary hearing; nor did he perform a neurological examination on Ms. Schiavo. He did, however, review Dr. Hammesfahr's extensive videotapes. Dr. Cheshire is on the Board of Directors of the Center for Bioethics and Culture and is a member of the Christian Medical Association's

Ethics Commission. Both these organizations ascribe to "Biblical values and principles." Judge Greer did not take his report seriously.

On the same day Dr. Cheshire submitted his report to the court, the Mayo Clinic also released a statement. "Mayo Clinic recognizes that the standard of care for the evaluation of a comatose patient includes a detailed review of the patient's history and previous evaluations as well as the performance of a comprehensive neurological examination. In some instances, electrophysiological and imaging studies may be used to establish a diagnosis." The Clinic's statement then added in the final paragraph, "Dr. Cheshire is not available for interviews."

Also on March 23, 2005, the American Academy of Neurology, the main national specialty society representing neurologists and a leader in the field of medical ethics, especially related to ethical issues involving patients with severe brain damage, issued a statement including the following point, "We have also reviewed the Congressional Record, articles in the media, and documents recently filed with the federal court. It appears that many public officials, representatives of the media, and others are ill-informed about the persistent vegetative state. Accordingly, the Academy leadership will be considering options for informing public officials, the media, and the public about the persistent vegetative state and the importance of preparing advance directives."[29]

:: The Medical Examiner's Report

This was the first major right-to-die case in which an autopsy was performed soon after the death of the patient to address directly the facts of the case and verify the neurological diagnosis. Dr. Jon Thogmartin, the medical examiner for Pinellas and Pasco counties, recognizing the great significance of his responsibilities, performed the most comprehensive and definitive autopsy and medical examiner's report that I have ever seen.[30] Dr. Thogmartin enlisted the expertise of numerous specialists around the country, including a forensic neuropathologist, Dr. Stephen Nelson.

The autopsy and conclusions of Dr. Thogmartin's report completely confirmed the clinical diagnosis of PVS. The brain, in both gross and microscopic examinations, showed extensive damage to the cerebral cortex, demonstrating profound hypoxic-ischemic encephalopathy. "Mrs. Schiavo's brain showed marked global anoxic-ischemic encephalopathy resulting in massive cerebral atrophy," the report said. This is exactly what the clinical experts said the brain would show at autopsy.[31] It continued: "Her brain weight was approximately half of the expected weight. Of particular importance was the hypoxic damage and neuronal loss in her occipital lobes, which indicates cortical blindness. Her remaining brain regions also show severe hypoxic injury and neuronal atrophy/loss."

During a news conference held at the time of the release of the medical examiner's report, Dr. Nelson noted that "persistent vegetative state . . . is a clinical diagnosis, it's not a pathologic diagnosis that has precision associated with it. . . . [but] There is nothing in her autopsy report, in her autopsy that is inconsistent with persistent vegetative state. . . . [data] are all are consistent with what is reported in the literature for persistent vegetative state."[32]

Dr. Thogmartin made it clear that no kind or amount of therapy would have helped: "This damage was irreversible. No amount of therapy or treatment would have regenerated the massive loss of neurons."[33] Thus the most important conclusion from the medical examiner's report was that Terri Schiavo had suffered a devastating and irreversible injury to the higher centers of the brain (the cerebral cortex) in 1990 and that she was never a candidate for any treatment to reverse this brain injury.

The vast majority of neurological specialists who are experienced and knowledgeable in the clinical and pathological findings of PVS, as well as most Americans who followed this case closely over the years, recognized the strong correlation between the clinical findings and the confirmatory findings at autopsy. It meant that the autopsy was the beginning of the end for those politicians who hoped to use the Schiavo case to advance their agenda: "WASHINGTON, June 15—The autopsy of Terri Schiavo—particularly the findings that she had irreversible brain damage and was blind—left Republicans who had pushed so aggressively for federal intervention struggling . . . to defend their argument that she should have been kept alive."[34]

∷ Eternal Denial?

On July 16, 2005, the Schindler family released a statement to the news media in response to the findings of the medical examiner's report.[35] Highlights include the following comments—with correcting annotations:

Our family stands by its strong belief that Terri was not in PVS, and we appreciate the many noted neurologists, including Dr. Cheshire who saw Terri just weeks before she died, who agree with our position.

We knew that Terri was visually impaired, but we did not know to what extent. Our attorneys and other witnesses clearly saw Terri recognize her mother and father and treat them differently. According to the IME's report, it appears that after her severe dehydration, Terri was blind at the moment of her death. [The medical examiner made it clear that Terri Schiavo was blind, completely blind, and not just visually impaired. The process of terminal dehydration had nothing whatsoever to do with the profound ischemic infarction of the visual cortex, which occurred at the time of the cardiac arrest on February 25, 1990, 15 years prior to the terminal dehydration in the last 13 days of Terri's life.]

Terri was brain-injured. This does NOT mean that she was brain-dead. Many seem to not understand this absolutely critical distinction. [No one ever knowingly said Ms. Schiavo was brain dead. Neither brain death nor the "crucial distinction" between "brain injured" and "brain dead" was ever an issue in this case—only the difference between being PVS or not.]

The IME's report stated that Terri's inability to swallow was the result of muscle atrophy. Terry was denied therapy for 12 years, and muscles atrophy when they are not used. We will never know if therapy would have helped. [The medical examiner's report unequivocally concludes that Ms. Schiavo's brain injury was irreversible. The inability to swallow was primarily due to the neurological condition, not due to any lack of therapy or any secondary atrophy of the neck or swallowing muscles.]

The medical facts of the case were thus and strongly rejected throughout and thereafter. Dr. Hammesfahr was the only one of eight neurologists who examined Ms. Schiavo and said she was definitely aware and responsive to commands, and could respond to medical treatment. His testimony and recommended form of medical treatment were, recall, completely rejected by Judge Greer. Dr. Hammesfahr issued a statement on the Christian Wire Service on June 19, 2005, in response to the medical examiner's report.[36] His remarks were in such direct conflict with mainstream medical opinion that it is difficult to address them. But let's try:

> Considering that there were so many physicians and therapists who were willing to step forward to treat Terri Schiavo, from university based practitioners to those in private practice, it clearly shows that the mainstream medical community across the board, those involved in treating patients, knew that they could help Terri.

> *To suggest the faulty affidavits represented the "mainstream medical community" is, simply, false. The opinions expressed in the affidavits not only were rejected by the courts but also were proved to be fallacious by outside neurologists and, ultimately, the results of the official autopsy.*

Obviously, the pathologists' comments that she could not see were not borne out by reality, and thus this assessment must represent sampling error.

The autopsy shows total bilateral destruction of the entire visual cortex (ischemic-infarction) by visual inspection. There was no "sampling error."

The autopsy results confirmed my opinion and Dr. Mayfield's opinions, that the frontal areas of the brains, the areas that deal with awareness and cognition were relatively intact.

The autopsy results completely refuted Dr. Hammesfahr's and Dr. Maxfield's views. Dr. Hammesfahr has taken Dr. Nelson's words "relatively intact" completely out of context. The entire cerebral cortex showed massive destruction with more extensive and observable destruction of the posterior areas of the brain. Under the microscopic section of the autopsy, Dr. Nelson notes: "The frontal and temporal poles and insular cortex demonstrated relative preservation" (compared to other, more extensively damaged areas). Further, the "frontal and temporal poles and insular cortex" are not areas of the brain that deal with awareness and cognition.

That she could not swallow was obviously not borne out by the reality that she was swallowing her saliva, about 1.5 liters per day of liquid.

It is a well-established fact that patients in a vegetative state can handle normal secretions by means of an intact involuntary swallowing reflex, and the fact that Ms. Schiavo could handle her own secretions is completely compatible with the diagnosis of the vegetative state.

Ultimately, based on the clinical evidence and the autopsy results, an aware woman was killed.

Surely this is politics, not medicine.

This extraordinary disconnect between medical fact and public utterance is worth documenting at length because of the prevalence of such views, and the lofty places they have reached. I do not know how to explain this phenomenon—but there is no doubt but that it must be documented and its consequences studied

∷ Conclusion

In the entire history of the right-to-die movement, there has never been a case in which such overwhelming and objective evidence was brought to bear, correlating the diagnosis of doctors who cared for a patient for 15 years, the opinions of credible medical experts testifying in court, the EEG, the neuroimaging studies, the opinions of the trial and appellate court judges who reviewed all the medical evidence in great detail, and, finally, the autopsy report.

In fact, the evidence could not have been more overwhelming: The EEG could not have been "flatter," the CT scan could have shown much more severe atrophy, and the examination of the brain post-mortem could hardly have shown much more significant brain damage. And the opinions of the opponents—including the observations of the Schindler family, the testimony of their medical experts at trial, the misleading videotapes released to the public, the flawed affidavits, and false beliefs and misguided opinions of the governor of Florida, leaders in the halls of Congress, and the president himself—could not have been more completely refuted than by this combination of clinical, laboratory, and pathology data.

The "Save Terri" partisans could not, and cannot, accept the medical facts of Ms. Schiavo's condition because, if they did, it would mean that their position was flawed from the beginning, and that all their efforts over 15 years were futile. Most Americans know now that Ms. Schiavo was in a PVS all along, but the conservatives will never be able to concede this medical fact. These opponents have been thoroughly discredited by the *Schiavo* case, as they should have been, having broken the first rule in law and ethics: Get your facts straight.

NOTES TO CHAPTER 6

1. Cranford, R.E. Facts, lies, and videotapes: The permanent vegetative state and the sad case of Terri Schiavo. *Journal of Law, Medicine & Ethics* 2005;33:363–371; Annas, G.J. "Culture of life" politics at the bedside—the case of Terri Schiavo. *New England Journal of Medicine* 2005;352:1710–1715; Quill, T.E. Terri Schiavo—a tragedy compounded. *New England Journal of Medicine* 2005;352:1630–1633.

2. American Academy of Neurology. Position of the American Academy of Neurology on Certain Aspects of the Care and Management of the Persistent Vegetative State Patient. *Neurology* 1989;39:125–126.; Ashwal, S., Cranford, R., Bernat, J.L., et al. (Multi-Society Task Force on PVS). Medical aspects of the persistent vegetative state—first of two parts. *New England Journal of Medicine* 1994;330:1499–1508, and Ashwal, S., Cranford, R., Bernat, J.L., et al. (Multi-Society Task Force on PVS). Medical aspects of the persistent vegetative state—second of two parts. *New England Journal of Medicine* 1994;330:1572–1579. (These statements were approved by the American Academy of Neurology, the Child Neurology Society, the American Academy of Pediatrics, the American Association of Neurological Surgeons, and the American Neurological Association.) See also Giacino, J., Ashwal, S., Childs, N., Cranford, R., et al. The

minimally conscious state: Definition and diagnostic criteria, *Neurology* 2002;58:349–353; Ashwal, S., and Cranford, R. The minimally conscious state in children. *Seminars in Pediatric Neurology* 2002;9:19–34; National Center of State Courts, Coordinating Council on Life-Sustaining Medical Treatment Decision Making by the Courts. *Guidelines for State Court Decision Making in Life-Sustaining Medical Treatment Cases,* revised 2nd edition. St. Paul: West Publishing Company, 1993.

3. *In re Schiavo* (Fla. Cir. Ct., February 11, 2000) (No. 90–2908-

4. GB-003), Judge George Greer. Available under the Timeline entry at February 11, 2000 at http://www.miami.edu/ethics/schiavo/schiavo_timeline.html

5. *In re Schiavo,* 780 So. 2d 176,177 (Fla. Dist. Ct. App. 2001), review denied 789 So. 2d 348 (Fla. 2001) (Schiavo I); see Cranford, "Facts, lies, and videotapes," pp. 365–366.

6. *In re Schiavo,* 2002 WL 31817960 (Fla. Cir. Ct. Nov. 22, 2002) (No. 90–2908-GB-003). Available under the Timeline entry for November 22, 2002, at http://www.miami.edu/ethics/schiavo/schiavo_timeline.html

7. Ibid., note 5, p. 7. Emphasis added. For a review of Dr. Hammesfahr's use of transcranial Doppler testing and vasodilator therapy, see the comments by Dr. Steven Novella on www.quackwatch.com, most recent revision February 14, 2000.

8. Ibid.

9. *In re Schiavo,* 851 So. 2d 182 (2nd DCA 2003) (No. 2D02–5394), *rehearing denied* (July 9, 2003), *review denied* 855 So. 2d 621 (Fla. 2003). Available under the Timeline entry for June 6, 2003, at http://www.miami.edu/ethics/schiavo/schiavo_timeline.html

10. Ibid.

11. Ibid.

12. *In re Schiavo,* 2002 WL 31817960 (Fla. Cir. Ct. Nov. 22, 2002) (No. 90–2908-GB-003). Available under the Timeline entry for November 22, 2002, at http://www.miami.edu/ethics/schiavo/schiavo_timeline.html

13. Alfonso, W.A., Lanting, D., Duenas, R.F., Cullen, and O. Papazian. Discontinuation of artificial hydration and nutrition in hopelessly vegetative children. *Annals of*

14. *Neurology* 1992;32:454–455. For the Brophy case, see *Brophy v. New England Sinai Hospital, Inc.,* 398 Mass. 417, 497 N.E.2d 626 (1986).

15. Eisenberg, J.B. *Using Terri: The Religious Right's Conspiracy to Take Away Our Rights.* New York: HarperCollins, 2005, p. 153. Eisenberg describes how DeLay in 1988 concurred in a family decision to take his father off life support.

16. Florida Bioethics Leaders' Commentary on HB701, March 7, 2005, Corrected 3–10. Available under the Timeline entry for March 7, 2005, at http://www.miami.edu/ethics/schiavo/schiavo_timeline.html.

17. Roberts, J., and Cranford, R.E. Terminal dehydration: The Deaths of Christine Busalacchi, Jamie Butcher, and Nancy Cruzan, unpublished manuscript.

18. Terrisfight.org, September 29, 2005. The "Report of Autopsy" by Jon R. Thogmartin, Chief Medical Examiner, District Six, Pasco & Pinellas

Counties, June 13, 2005, is available under the timeline entry for June 15, 2005, at http://www.miami.edu/ethics/schiavo/schiavo_timeline.html.

19. Wolfson, J. Erring on the side of Theresa Schiavo: Reflections of the
20. special guardian ad litem. *Hastings Center Report* 2005;35(3):16–19.
21. *Congressional Record*, 109th Cong., 1st sess, 2005, Vol. 151, pt. 26:H993 (March 8). This and subsequent citations from the *Congressional Record* are available at http://www.gpoaccess.gov/crecord/index.html.
22. Ibid.
23. *Congressional Record*, 109th Cong., 1st sess., 2005, Vol. 151, pt. 32:H1601 (March 16).
24. Ibid.
25. *Congressional Record*, 109th Cong., 1st sess, 2005, Vol. 151, pt. 33, Book II:S3091 (March 17).
26. Eisenberg, *Using Terri*, p. 202.
27. 24. CNN.com. Frist knocks Edwards over stem cell comment. CNN, October 12, 2004. Available at http://www.cnn.com.
28. Rich, F. In the beginning, there was Abramoff. *The New York Times*, October 2, 2005, p. 12.
29. Declaration of Barbara J. Weller, Appendix 7 to emergency motion by the Schindlers to have Judge Greer remove her tube. Available on the Web under the March 26, 2005, Timeline entry at http://www.miami.edu/ethics/schiavo.
30. Letter by Dr. Stephen J. Nelson as attachment to "Report of Autopsy" (see note 16).
31. Affidavit, State of Florida, County of Duval, William Polk Cheshire, MD, MA, FACP, March 23, 2005. Available on the Web under the March 23, 2005, timeline entry at http://www.miami.edu/ethics/schiavo.
32. Mayo Clinic in Jacksonville, Florida, March 23, 2005, Comment on Dr. William Cheshire's involvement with Department of Children and Families; Statement of American Academy of Neurology, March 23, 2005, released from the Academy headquarters in Minneapolis, Minnesota, by Sandra Olson, current President of AAN; available at www.aan.com. Cf. the Mayo Clinic's news release at http://www.mayoclinic.org/news2005-jax/2724.html
33. "Report of Autopsy."
34. Ibid., p. 8, #6.
35. Johnson, J. Terri Schiavo autopsy: Manner of death "undetermined." CNSNews.com June 15, 2005. Note that the phrases "permanent vegetative state" and "persistent vegetative state" are sometimes and incorrectly used interchangeably. See Cranford, R. Diagnosing the permanent vegetative state. American Medical Association Virtual Mentor, August 2004, http://www.ama-assn.org/ama/pub/category/12720.html. For an important early perspective, see Jennet, B., and Plum, F. Persistent vegetative state after brain damage; a syndrome in search of a name. *Lancet* 1972;1:734–737.
36. Goodnough, A. Schiavo autopsy says brain, withered, was untreatable. *The New York Times*, June 16, 2005. Available at http://www.nyt.com.

37. Kornblut, A.E. Schiavo autopsy renews debate on G.O.P. actions. *The New York Times*, June 16, 2005. Available at http://www.nyt.com.
38. Schindler Family's Statement on Medical Examiner's Report, issued June 16, 2005. Available on the Web under that date in the Timeline at http://www.miami.edu/ethics/schiavo.
36. Christian Communication Network. Physician who examined Schiavo for over 10 hours critical of autopsy report. Christian Wire Service, June 19, 2005. http://www.earnedmedia.org/

7 ::

Crossing the Borderlands at Nightfall: New Issues in Moral Philosophy and Faith at the End of Life

Laurie Zoloth

:: Border Crossings at Nightfall I: Death and Transgression

There was a time in the spring of 2005, the week of Passover and Easter, as it happened, when all there was to talk about was the case of Mrs. Terri Schiavo. We spoke about her as if we knew her, casually calling her "Terri" and arguing about her marriage and how her mother touched her face, as if it were our business (which, of course, if you were a bioethicist, it oddly was), her image cast before our gaze on 24-hour news shows, on pop talk shows. It was on the TV in the airport, on the front page of every newspaper. It was on TV when I checked into a tiny motel in North Carolina, and the nightshift desk clerk and I, the Baptist and the Jewish traveler, watched for hours on the night that the United States Congress debated the issue, improbably, into the early morning. We saw brain scans that were posted (HIPAA rules notwithstanding) on the Internet. We talked about advance directives and surrogates with strangers on elevators and checkout lines and, suddenly, the obscuranta of bioethics was vividly displayed: this idea that families could withdraw treatment and allow their loved ones to die was a staple of our work, but here we were, with the entire process broken down, failed, on national television, and the idea itself was challenged. This was what it would mean to die publicly. We stood before the endless loop of tape, the baby and childhood pictures of this woman, and she was in each living room, dying. One could not turn away from that thing that all humans know but suppress: I am vulnerable, just like that, utterly dependent on the mercy of others, and then I will die. It is the ultimately normal, yet utterly transgressive act—the interruption of being and of time itself.

Three framing issues: What sort of a question should we be asking about this case?

First: Publicity and Presence

Why is death a *public* bioethical issue at all, and why is death a public *bioethical* issue at all? Why indeed is death the subject of so many national conferences on bioethics, as opposed to, for example, vaccine policies, or environmental public health, or foster care? Why would the most fundamental reality of a human life—that, finally, we all are born, that we all die, and that we do this one by one—be the subject of our public gaze and our controversy? Is this great public attention, even this chapter, in even this volume, simply the bioethicist's version of the media tent at the bedside in the Schiavo case, framing and abstracting, and, finally, even selling the case?[1] If, as Peter Berger reminds us, it is religion that erects the great tent of mercy and meaning in the face of death, how did bioethics achieve the status of guardian of our borders of death? Or the erector of this sort of sacred canopy at all?[2]

It was the nature of moral philosophy to ask the question, "What does it mean to *live* a good life?"[3] In this way, of course, we debated death as a surrogate for this larger, more contentious question—is your life worth it? In bioethics, such a question turned toward death and its management, as opposed to moral behavior, just aspirations, or the fittingness of one's work. We do not, largely, ask: On behalf of what sort of actions should we be arguing to aim us toward a good, or ethical life? We asked, rather, only about the managerial question of when it was permissible to refuse care that might keep us alive. It became the nature of bioethics and health care policy to then ask: Is your care worth paying for, or worth devoting resources toward? This sort of question yielded nicely to details about the sort of machines that performed the care, and charts about feeding tubes, or respirators, or electrical paddles. Thus began the institutionalization of "futility policies" in which hospitals could make such a decision unilaterally, and the legal, even written, contracts, signed in advance, and linked, not surprisingly, to Medicare payment options, about hospice vs. ICU care, and other end-of-life directions given in advance.

Second: Patterns of Meaning

The one-year anniversary of this case provided the distance to see patterns of meaning and of social consequence in the event . . . and this very sentence leads me to stop and think about the act of sequence and sentencing itself, the turning into language, and, worse, into a mercantile exchange, the tragedy of the death of a stranger as something that can be abstracted, then packaged up, then bought and sold.

It is clear that each new case recasts the discourse about end-of-life decision making—this has been true since Karen Ann Quinlan's doctors first testified that they believed parents had no right or expertise to withdraw care. These public acts of death and dying created a shifting consensus about medicine at the end of life. A year after the Schiavo case, the number of people who supported the decision—63 percent—changed only a percentage point, to 64 percent. More than a quarter of Americans opposed the withdrawal of the feeding tube,[4] and who they represent is interesting, for it is not only the religious right who oppose treatment withdrawal, it is also patient advocacy and disability rights groups[5] that had previously supported it. In other words, opposing medicine itself leads now to wanting (paradoxically) more aggressive medical care; opposing the decision of doctors to act as the border patrol at death's frontier now means switching sides in a longstanding debate over the right to die (think here on the play and film "Whose Life Is It Anyway?", which took the opposite position). Further, the ability to visualize and image the brain, and the capacity for far more effective rehabilitative medicine, led to two opposing tensions in American life. Hence, the advances in neuroscience restructured the American response to death but in opposite directions: For some, they provided a certainty about the idea of irreversibility, but for others, they provided a scaffold for an unlimited hope, precisely, of reversal.

Final Point: Humility and Cases

Let me plead for some humility in this, even as we speak here, out of our vast unknowing and our seeming know-it-all stance. Bioethicists were in the news in a way that was unprecedented, telling us what this death meant. At the national level, Caplan, Charo, and Cranford were interviewed on television, Emanuel was on NPR, several others, this author included, were in *The New York Times* and *The Washington Post*, and in every newspaper in every town with a university, bioethicists were called forward. We did, as a field, fairly decent work, in this instance calling on all families to reflect in advance on the issues. Bioethics became a part of the story, for in part the case was about expertise itself, and about our own yearning for permission and rules. Informed consent and the theory of law, beloved of bioethicists, were challenged, and many bioethicists worried aloud that "our" entire framework of how we made these decisions would be undone by this case. The case created its own schedule, as faculty in the law, journalism, and medicine all were drawn into debate. I received bewildered calls from reporters who said, in essence, "I really haven't a clue about this medical stuff, I usually just cover Congress," as the debate moved into the House and Senate. As a field, bioethicists had expertise in cases like this: Many scholars and practitioners of clinical ethics consultation had experience with families in the sort of persistent denial/hopefulness that Mrs. Schiavo's case seem to display, and had known spouses who, after years of valiant caregiving, began to change their minds and sought the end of care they learned would not change the situation of their loved ones—spouses seeming to reverse course, as Mr. Schiavo had done.

Yet, really, like everyone, we bioethicists were far from the role that we usually insist on in clinical work—first-hand knowledge of the case. We participated in our distant analysis, as much as the field of bioethics was critical of the congressional long-distance video diagnostics. Even in the faith communities that were called upon to comment on The Case, there was a sense of involvement in the intensity of the case that displayed the curious nature of the event—in part symbolic, in part performance of some larger discourse, a compelling and tangible and immediate "text" that drew one away from ordinary ethical duties and realities. One early morning, I found myself walking along Michigan Avenue, listening to a radio show to debate The Case, passing a row of beggars, ironically, with signs just like the ones in Florida—"Feed me" and "Hungry" lettered on gray cardboard in the rain—and wondered why the radio station wasn't having a show on the problem of hunger and homeless strangers on their doorstep, why Jesse Jackson and the clergy, and the crowds of praying people, and the Congressmen, and the reporters, much less the bioethicists, were not right here, offering food and care. Everyone was in Florida. There was no gaze on Mrs. Schiavo that did not use her, thematize her, mark her as ours. As a nation, America spoke of her, she who had become "The Case," as an episode in their own lives, her death some personal event. There "was no family spared this death," for it was shown (unsparingly) every hour, in one's kitchen, in one's living room, and, weirdly enough, between commercials.

:: Border Crossings at Nightfall II: Faith and Death

29. And it came to pass, that at midnight the Lord struck all the firstborn in the land of Egypt, from the firstborn of Pharaoh who sat on his throne to the firstborn of the captive who was in the dungeon; and all the firstborn of cattle.

30. And Pharaoh rose up in the night, he, and all his servants, and all the Egyptians; and there was a great cry in Egypt; for there was not a house where there was not one dead.

31. And he called for Moses and Aaron by night, and said, Rise up, and get out from among my people, both you and the people of Israel; and go, serve the Lord, as you have said.

32. Also take your flocks and your herds, as you have said, and be gone; and bless me also.

33. And the Egyptians urged the people, that they might send them out of the land in haste; for they said, We shall all be dead men.

What is occurring here? It is the re-telling into action of what has been promised as the final plague on Pharaoh, told to Moses so that he, in the face of this terrible death of his neighbors, can prepare the Hebrew slaves to survive by participation in the Passover ceremony. Pharaoh, understanding at last, despite his impossibly hardened capacity for mercy, that loss and chaos touches everyone "for there was not a house where there was not one dead," allows the Jews to leave to go worship God, at last. This is the fundamental core of the Exodus narrative, the central problem in three religious, Abrahamic traditions of Judaism, Christianity, and Islam. It is a text about the complex relationship between death, faith, and liberation. For a scholar who reads the Biblical text, the phrase is a familiar one: the description of the shared event of death of the beloved child, the night before liberation, the "dead one" in every house, is read, of course, in the season of Passover and Easter. Hence, there was no way to separate entirely the apprehension of this death from the apprehension of the approach of the holidays and their rich and multivocal evocations of death and miracle.

The way this death was then witnessed and "worded" allowed everyone to make such metaphors (as I just did) to thematize and prove their point, which was often a point about belief. Nancy Grace, CNN's legal reporter, lead the discourse of those who saw this as a version of the Killer Husband Narrative, with Mrs. Schiavo cast as Laci Peterson. The elegant, grieving Joan Didion saw her as her own dying daughter and wrote of this extensively in *The New York Review of Books*. Indeed, the adult woman, Mrs. Schiavo, became the face of vulnerability and sacrifice itself, struck down in the middle of the dark of night, as in the Hebrew Scripture, the desexualized child to many, dressed in her frilly nightgown like Wendy in a "Peter Pan" play, virginal, her face a mask of perfect innocence. She was shown in her communion dress, in her white wedding gown, a permissible possession for the discourse within faith communities.

A woman in an irreversible coma enters into a category of our making, a new terrain tractable only if rescue is possible, nursing care is excellent, and funding for intensive care is plentiful. Such a women is utterly dependent on a complex culture and community and economy, not just the machines. She is, of course, not dead, in that she cycles in and out of fertility and makes insulin, and her heart beats and she breathes. We understand that the physical place of her mind has been destroyed; she is an object of our compassion—but an object, no longer the subject of her own life. Ironically, she is entirely embodied, in that she has no capacity for consciousness, no phenomenological or narrative or subjective being. Yet the actual embodied details of care—the menstrual periods, the bowel movements, the care of her PEG tube, the contractures of her hands and spine, what it takes to care for such a body—are not a part of the way she is portrayed, for she is curiously disembodied, in this way as well.

There were hundreds of medical details, etiologies of illness, neuroscientific facts, and nursing histories to know about The Case, and one could argue fruitlessly about data that became steadily useless against the one thing that people could see: the tape of her seemingly watching eyes, and seemingly pleased smile. Unlike Quinlan's and other cases, this story could be witnessed and the ubiquitous reportage re-witnessed.

The Culture of the Partaking Witness

It is not only the technology that transmitted the narrative that had changed, but the culture. Quinlan, Cruzan, and Wendland are names that mean something to people who study bioethics, but little to others who do not learn the history of treatment withdrawal. However, because news is now both 24 hours and shown worldwide, this dying, this image, became a symbol of American discourse itself and was front-page news all over the world. (A particular oddity, especially when that spring, so many were dying: in the Sudan, in Iraq, in Romania.)

It is my contention it did so in the larger culture in part because it occurred just as Americans were having three other struggles about borders, families, and death that were harder to visualize, struggles *qua* debates that affected our sense of order and permission in *this* case. American borders, our relationships with the outside world, and the "brokenness of borders" shape the language of modernity itself. The first of these was that after 9/11, in which American borders were suddenly broached, the ideas of death and chance and risk were altered. People were trying to kill you—this is now the message of every plane trip, of every search of your bag at the baseball park. Moreover, Americans were at war, a war that, for the first time since Vietnam, seemed circular at best, resisting all linear attempts at cause-and-effect narrative; at beginning, middle, and end; or at final resolutions, despite technological superiority. In the case of the Afghan and Iraqi aspects of the war, the photos of dead young sons and daughters were not shown—the very opposite of the Schiavo case.

Second, Americans were also having a debate about the borders of the natural. Many of the forces that aligned in the case on the issue of death and dying surfaced in other debates about modernity and technology. Here, religious traditions used the entrance into life (embryos, stem cells, abortion) and the exit from it (withdrawal of medical care, brain death criteria) as surrogates for moral concern about human intervention into processes understood as "natural" and also as sacred, or supernatural, in the control, properly, of God.

Third, Americans were also having a debate about the borders of family life and the nature or authority of the state to define and legislate it. This largely took the form, in that year, of whether gay marriage was permissible, and if so, what role the state should have in the matter, but it was also a continuation of a longer debate about marriage itself, so the virginal, white church wedding of the Schiavos was depicted against the common-law marriage of Mr. Schiavo to his second wife,[6] their children, their home, where they washed the clothes of Mrs. Schiavo.

Death and the Nightly News

It was not the first time that modernity and technology and war coincided with images of death. In fact, the birth and first widespread use of photography itself was to witness the corpses of the War Between the States. The Civil War was fought in the center of towns, just as new technology reshaped the American terrain—trains, rapid repeating rifles, and civil engineering created a new sort of death, and the use of death masks and the reprinting of the faces and bodies of the newly, violently dead made the death itself invasive. Oddly, the first battles of the Civil

War were witnessed by picnickers as well, until the carnage and chaos overtook them—hence the photographs. The witness to dying was a feature of modernity. Yet in this, too, Christians were able to see and understand the witness of death as an echo of the Cross—a fact inescapably made in the signs and banners of the witnessing protestors outside the hospice in Florida.

Desacralization and Modernity

It is this tension between the desacralization of death (in every home; on the news hourly between commercials) and the private re-sacralization of the normative hospital experience (praying crowds and crosses) that drew communities of faith so profoundly into the personal yet public occasion of this particular death.

The idea of religion in America is linked to freedom. It includes, then, an idea of a space, normally protected by family and ties of love, of a relationship (both a duty and a liberation) that was outside the adjudication of the state in that any particular kind or type of relationship, including a skepticism about the very project itself, could be freely chosen without prohibition by the government. Yet Americans, despite increasing diversity in religious choices,7 are largely varieties of Christians. In thinking about religion and the meaning of death, it is important to remember that in all the cases of witnessed public death cases (Quinlan was the paradigm) the actual issue is not one of "religion" but of American Christian faith—in Quinlan and Schiavo, Roman Catholic faith—as lived in a Protestant Christian country that over three decades became a far more fervently religious country in which public displays of religiosity were increasingly common. The religious question at stake was, "How does a Christian die?"

It is true that all religion addresses the issue of suffering and the meaning of life in the face of contingency, but it was the particular attention to and theological response to the problem of death—featuring the killing and resurrection of the leader understood as divine, allowing the possibility of a life after death, and creating a richly imagined and fully established heaven, limbo, purgatory, and hell as the venue for that afterlife—that gave Christianity much of its distinctiveness, its authority, and its normative power. Religious Jews, Hindus, Buddhists, and Muslims apprehend the questions of death differently—hence, at issue here was in part a church–state controversy as well.

Further, earlier discussions about the moment of death and treatment withdrawal were inflected by the use of organs for transplantation.

Discussion of treatment withdrawal in cases like Mrs. Schiavo's raised two different sorts of issues. First, what was the status of persons in persistent vegetative states, and did that diagnosis make us more or less duty-bound to respect their wishes and advanced verbal directives? Second, was there something unique about the withdrawal of artificial nutrition and hydration, linked as it was to religious texts about the moral gesture of offering food and water to guests? This gesture is the central act of faith in several texts in the Hebrew scripture, the New Testament, and the Koran, and, as in the other cases of treatment withdrawal—Cruzan, Wendland, Draybeck—such a gesture has prompted a renegotiation with the texts. How much could the state adjudicate in cases of rights for persons in liminal status, when religions differed on the issue so deeply? Yet, how could traditions turn from an increasingly common question, now that nursing care and ICU rescue began to create entire new categories of being? Finally, the witnessing of this death of a Christian, on Holy Week, which was followed by the witnessing of the death of the Pope (*The* Christian, to many, and surely to the Catholic families who were most deeply identified with the Schiavo case), meant that many faith communities were called to reflect on the particularities of response—both about how to be a witness to this Christian death, and how to understand the right way for a Jew to die, or a Muslim, or an atheist for that matter. The case was debated in Israel, for example, and the Knesset passed new laws widening permission to withdraw care.

In 1973, as Catherine Belling notes,[7] not only was the Quinlan case first recasting the issue of death as strategy, but the novel *Coma* was being written. In *Coma*, the novel and the movie, the reader encountered a new sort of human possibility, what Belling calls "the living dead," invoking the horror movie of the same name. In the fictional account, the comas are induced deliberately, there is foul play, and the bodies are sought for their organs. This theme was then introduced in film images—floating, young bodies—not quite corpses, not quite sleeping, for they entirely depended on technology to keep them alive. The technology is vital; the tube to the pump is key. In later years, the fictional narrative began to mirror the medical one. In movies, two separate categories began to merge in the public mind: the liminal status of the comatose patient (here one thinks of Mrs. Schiavo's mother saying, "But she is perfectly healthy, all she is is brain damaged") and the liminal status of the newly created and then frozen embryo. Any Buddhist or Hindu scholar could tell us that death is not the opposite of life, but of birth,[8] and any film scholar would make the same point.[9] When the activities of birth are disaggregated (as in modern assisted reproductive technology), a new category of dependent being is created, and when the activities of death are disaggregated and deconstructed (as in the modern ICU), a similarly new category of dependent being is created. Then, what is at stake is our duties toward the dependent being we have—or rather the new technology that we wield, pay for, and support has—created.

Thus it was clear, outside the Schiavo hospice, that the two liminal states of being had merged into one controversy, that of the "right to life." It was true for the Pope, who had commented on the case and written extensively about the "seamless network of life" and the theological link among contingent, vulnerable beings; his own simultaneous death would finally end the broadcast of the story. It was true for the demonstrators, and later, in the literature that followed, liminality, moral status, withdrawal of care, and embryos became deeply intertwined. The very same year that Americans debated the Schiavo case, the President's Council on Bioethics embarked on a plan to define and create embryos that did not have the moral status of embryos, and at one point used the example of brain death criteria as a template for this moral argument.

For the Catholic Church, however, the insistence on the impermissibility of treatment withdrawal was not always the case. Medieval Church writings warn against the fear of doctors overtreating, or of overconfidence in medicine.[10] In fact, earlier work on the Quinlan case by Catholic moral theologians refined a classic consideration within the Church, that of "ordinary versus extraordinary treatment," in which only ordinary treatment was mandated, and thus, much of ICU care could be withdrawn. As ICU care and ventilators became increasingly ordinary, the Church expanded its reasoning to consider the weight of the burdens and benefits of treatment, including nutrition and hydration. In 1991, Jesuit bioethicist Richard McCormick wrote in favor of treatment withdrawal, basing his reflections on this "proportionality" guideline:

> Many ethicists and physicians are convinced that artificial nutrition and hydration are not required for persons diagnosed as irreversibly in a PVS. They base this view on the judgment that continuation in a PVS is not a benefit to the patient and therefore is not in the patient's best interest. This is my own conviction and I wrote as much in support of Lester and Joyce Cruzan's deacon to stop Nancy's gastrostomy feedings. Others, however—a minority, I believe—view this decision in much more sinister terms.[11]

Other Jesuits, including John Paris and John Golenski, expressed the need to interpret Catholic doctrines about treatment withdrawal for the PVS patient as permissive. James Bresnahan noted in 1991, as hospitals and other health care institutions receiving federal funds were required by the Patient Self Determination Act to provide information about advanced directives, that Catholics ought indeed to understand and accept dying as a part of the Christian story, becoming "graced in freedom in submission to death."[12] Thinking in advance about death and suffering, he argued, was precisely what was called for by Catholic theology and praxis—it was modern medical centers that created a medical culture that faith needed to question:

> Indeed, in my experience, the success of contemporary medicine in giving us "more time" often, if not always, brings with it the burden of a more difficult and frequently more painful dying.[13]

While many of these same scholars repeated their stands in 2005, addressing the Schiavo case, the Church's position had shifted. Despite calls by John Paris and others to attend to the earlier consensus and scholarship on the problem of suffering and the grace of a fitting and timely treatment withdrawal, the "minority voices" noted by McCormick in 1991 had become the dominant ones in the Church.

In Israel and in the Muslim world, new reflections on technology led in the opposite direction. One found the interpretations of tradition allowing increasing instances of treatment withdrawal. The debate in Israel was largely centered around the methodology of how to withdraw treatment without violation of the *halacha*, or Jewish religious laws that differentiate between the permissibility of treatment withholding (in cases where treatment was noncontinuous or newly initiated) and impermissibility (in cases where treatment was continuously offered). The Steinberg commission offered a creative solution—placing all patients on ventilators on timers that would interrupt the treatment to allow for moral reconsideration about the nature, goal, and meaning of the care.[14]

Hence the case began to emerge less as a reflection of religious differences than as a reflection of emerging political inflections in religious traditions within the new American context of religion, ethics, and public life. There were distinctive new turns in the case, one being the discourse among feminists, about fidelity, in which a vocal minority framed the debate in terms of the marriage; or of speculation about the cause of the initial anoxic insult, untreated potassium imbalances secondary to severe bulimic dieting patterns by Mrs. Schiavo; another, the calls of unfairness and discrimination by the disability rights community.

How should we credit these claims within the larger structures of religion? What moral appeals ought ethicists within religious traditions consider; what narratives will testify in this genre of case (since narratives are largely the method of religious ethics)? Let us turn to another story, for it may remind us of how our view of death and our first years of response to this problem have led us to this point. It is an account of a case far "easier" in the standard frames of bioethics, yet one that is instructive for the harder case we collectively faced in 2005.

The Easy Case: Spring 1992
A narrative:

When the chair of the ethics committee called, she was only slightly apologetic. "When you were away," she said, "we did an interesting case; it was easy, actually. I mean, it was terribly sad, but we knew what to do." She stopped, then was quiet. "Really, it was sad, but it was just like the ones we know well, that we studied, a classic treatment withdrawal case." I had been celebrating Passover and had not been on call for the case. We agreed to meet the next day, and when I walked into her office, she handed me a small package, brown wrapper, fresh cellophane tape. It was a video that the patient, Mr. C—the "case"—had made to show the ethics committee. The committee chair had neatly written the case up: withdrawal from a ventilator, the family and the doctor all agree, no contest.

She was right, of course. It was an easy case, it was like a hundred you can read about in which a patient is suddenly snatched from a vivid life into our intensive care unit: It is a fire, it is a heart attack, it is a fever, and this time it was a jump into a country swimming hole, a flight enjoyed often during this man's life. But this one time it landed him flat in bed, broken at the high neckline, C-4, the breath on that leap his last unassisted one.

"Doing a case" means that the ethics committee of the hospital, and it was a thoughtful one, listened carefully to the ethical dilemma, talked about the competing moral appeals, and reflected on various options, recommending one option to the family and the team. This happened nearly every week in that hospital, and here was another recommendation to support a patient and a family, no surprise, who wanted treatment to be withdrawn.

I watched the video at home that night, with my children asleep next to me, small reddish palms of babies in the light of the video, which is grainy, an old home video flickering over their sleeping faces. In it a man faces the camera, which is held by his wife who speaks to him and asks him the questions that the chair of the ethics committee has given her: Why do you want to stop the ventilator? Do you know you will die if we take the ventilator away? Are you depressed?

In a way I feel ashamed—the intrusiveness of the questions, the permission to see him like this, his need to convince us, the strangers who he must imagine beyond his wife's own face, and the terrible blank, unblinking stare of the camera.

He wants to die because we have failed him and he cannot imagine a life beyond this one we have given him, and he yearns for his old life back, a thing we call denial. We cannot stop his pain very well, he hates his passivity, he is a quadriplegic, and that is who he has become, his name—"the quad," "the case"—and he would rather be dead.

Principles and Practices in Bioethics

How could we have gotten to this place, where such a decision could be seen as easy, a straightforward right? Bioethics in 1992 had emerged just this far. We understood that of all the things we could do that would be of use, teaching the concept of ethical principle (beneficence, non-maleficence, justice, and autonomy) might be the most important. And of these, since the complex, well-intentioned power of the doctors really was (impressively) to do medical good, autonomy—the very power that could also be misused, the right of refusal—was what we taught as a core principle. We taught that against the power of the doctor, researcher, state, institution, church, or tradition, a patient could say "no" and that "no" would stand—even if everyone else thought that the treatment was needed. It would be the patient who would decide, the freely choosing, freely refusing patient who would know her own mind and her own creaturely limits best and be trusted and empowered to speak on her own behalf.

It was, initially, a contentious business, a matter for the courts at first, in Quinlan, Saikewicz, Herbert and Drabick and Bouvia, and the courts anguished about each sort of patient, each level of consciousness, each type of treatment that could be withheld. At a time in which civil rights, then human rights, were explored and expanded, bioethics fought what John Fletcher described as a battle[15] in which the line between analysis and advocacy, which nearly always meant advocacy for less intensive treatment, was often blurred.

This narrative paralleled the narrative of hospice care. Initial hospice meetings were often full of former ICU or NICU nurses who had simply had enough of invasive medical treatment as well—they wanted to withdraw treatment, and in the cases that they brought to the ethics committees, they spoke of how too much treatment could be harmful. They too stood behind the concept of the right to withdraw treatment at the patient's request. As an ethicist, I, too, was intent on learning the lessons of witness, of listening.

And thus we struggled to get DNR order forms into the hands of patients, we taught the staff to listen to patients. We helped to create a moral location—the ethics committee—that allowed for a serious moral discussion to occur. We did what the theologians suggested: allow such discussion to occur when patients faced difficult news, supporting the conversations about death and dying and advocating that patients be allowed to make treatment refusal decisions in advance of illness or injury, by an act of imagination.

Moral Imagination and Literature

It was an effort that was reflected in literature. In her story, "Compassion," writer Dorothy Allison relates the families' view of our attempts. Here, she writes about the nurse, Mavis.

> That evening, Mavis stopped me in the hall. She had a stack of papers in one hand and an expression that bordered on outrage. "This ain't been signed," she said. Her hand shook the papers. I looked at them as she stepped in close to me. She pulled one off of the bottom. "Look at this. Look at it close." The printing was dark and bold. "Do not resuscitate. No extraordinary measures to be taken." I looked up at Mavis and she shook her head at me. "Don't tell me you don't know what I mean. You been on this road a long time. You know what's coming, and your mother needs you to take care of it." She pressed a sheaf of papers into my hands. "You go in there and take another long look at your mother and then you get these papers done right."[16]

The ICU is a prison of sorts in this story, and we who have worked there understood this, and hence worked out a sort of subversive praxis between the intensity and necessity of modernity and the fragility of the bruised and contained love packed into the place. In the story, the narrator's mother begs to her daughters to let her smoke, and:

> Finally, Jo gave me a sharp look and we stood up as one. She went over to try to force the window open, pounding the window frame till it came loose. I dug around in Jo's purse, found her Marlboros, lit one, and held it to Mama's lips. Jo went and stood guard by the door. Mama coughed, sucked and smiled gratefully. "Baby," she whispered and fell asleep with ashes on her neck. Jo walked over and took the cigarette I still held. "Stupid damn

rules," she said bitterly. Mavis came in then, sniffed loudly and shook her head at me. "You know you can't do that." . . . I saw Mama's face smoothed. Her fingers in mine clutched tightly. "That window isn't supposed to be open," Mavis said suddenly. "You get it shut."[17]

To give her mother what is needed as she lies dying, the sisters must literally claw loose the framing apparatus of the window, and of the ICU itself; they must violate the orders not to touch their mother, who is in isolation for herpes; they must stay after hours; all of which is amplified by the subversion of the nurse. The mother asks each daughter in turn: What happens when you die?

I'm afraid. She gripped my hand so tightly I could feel the bones of my fingers rubbing together. "I know," I told her. "But I am here. I won't go anywhere. I'll stay right here."[18]

Finally, at her death, even the last daughter is "right there"—even the one who desperately hopes for a cure until the end.

I knew then. Arlene would go on as long as it took, making that sound in her throat like some bird creature, the one that comes to sing hope when there is no hope left. Strength was in Arlene's song, peace its meter, love the bass note . . . Mama's whole attention remained fixed on that song until the pupil of her right eye finally filled up with blood and blacked out. Even then we held on. We held Mama's stilled shape between us. We held her until she set us free.[19]

It is the setting free into death that creates an alternate conclusion to the tragic life described under the lines of the story, and the paradox that the arduous dying is the thing that allows for love at last is the ordinary miracle of the hospice. It was nurses like the Mavis of the story, who, finally weary of subversion, left the Unit to create this ordinary miracle outside the hi-tech venue—the hospice that would be the setting for Cruzan and Schiavo.

But so doing inevitably created a split in medical care—in which patients and families were actually asked to choose an opt-out path, widely understood as "giving up" by many. As the hospice movement grew in sophistication, it, not ICU, became the recipient of some of the best knowledge of palliation, pain control, and psychological support.

Is it really any wonder, then, that our "cases" seemed to feel such despair? It is in fact painful even to watch this video of the Easy Case, to wait for each sentence between the machine's sighing. The man in the video asked for death, and it seemed entirely logical, given this history, given the narrative we shaped about machines, about "the good death."

Mr. C was, moreover a religious man, and he believed in and spoke of an afterlife, but he largely made his case because he had asked the question, "Is this a life worth living?" and thought not. "I am a hands-on guy," he says, forlornly. "I can't wash the car, I can't mow the lawn." He seems quite clear, and he says he is not depressed, just "in a prison, here."

Yet, after watching, I told my colleague I thought they had made a mistake, and she shook her head; she was surprised. Why would I say such a thing?

Why indeed? I could not fully articulate why, for the case did indeed fit neatly within the parameters we all agreed were important. Yet, a year later, I found out—having asked permission to use this tape in teaching, a thing I do with discomfort each time (how can such a practice be permissible?). One of the nurses in the class began to cry. And so it turned out that there was more to the story, which surely renders it not so "easy." She had been the nurse on the case, and she had been unable to help her patient. The rules of the HMO had been rigid— he did not qualify for a motorized wheelchair, nor for rigorous therapies she had tried to fight for, the pain control they wanted to try was "off formulary" and difficult to obtain—in short, she told the class, *we do not know who he could have been if he had gotten all the care he needed.*

Hence, I began to wonder: Had we gone too far in our thinking about autonomy and end-of-life cases? Had we been so taken by liberty interests, by autonomy claims, that we had not seen the issue of justice clearly enough, or had turned from beneficence and some duties beyond erogatory ones? I always think of the flickering image on the tape (he is always a young man, my age when the tape was made, in 1990, yet I steadily age) and wonder: What was that death really about? In the years since, I have thought a great deal about this case. I have wondered what we ought to say to the man who only wants to escape us. Have we given up too easily? What would it mean to ask a broader question: How can medicine itself be transformed?—not, How can bioethics help patients escape from it? It would be to think about duties toward the transformation, and not the thinner demand of only one of the key rights, that of negation. Would that return us to the deeper question of beneficence—*how* is it that we do good? How can we transform the way to perform medicine into a place in which alternative strategies are normative?

It is not a new idea, it is merely a difficult idea, and that is because we collectively believe in, and have faith in, the technology to heal. We believe in the engineered solution, and in large part the belief is rewarded with survival. Patients come to the ICU betting they will live, and they put their bodies on the table, as it were, all that they have, willing for anything. To get to hospice, they must call off the bet. But what makes the movie of our case, the enactment of the consensual argument of bioethics so disturbing, is that we become accomplices in the death itself—and by so doing, we endorse the allocation decisions that force the choice. In this way, we play with the house, we are the house. Have we asked the question of justice carefully enough when we seek the answer of freedom?

It was in response to that sort of question that Ira Byock and many others have been working for years to reconfigure the entire scenario. Could even ICU care, the heart of it, be, simply, kinder? Could the kindness simply be part of the practice, not a resistant act? This is not to note the critical importance of resistant acts—to be sure, the bioethics community focused on this method, and on building a hermeneutical circle to critique medicine; and rightly so. We are devoted to this critique, which is why, in part, we hear and we understand the project of negation better than we have sympathy for the project of asking for more. In fact, when patients ask for what we perceive as "too much," they are marked as problematic, perhaps seeking treatment named to be futile. We understood the call for hospice care, and for treatment withdrawal of all kinds. The hospice was widely understood as the place of compassion and expertise. And one could argue that the logic of the end-of-life movement and our commitment to it is largely a victory. We thought about how the wider social world shapes the intense internal world of the ICU, and wrote policies that began a process of reform even there. New guidelines for pain and palliation have begun to be a part of how all patients are assessed, and all patients and families are confronted with advance directive forms and conversations about death and the careful choosing of a surrogate decision-maker.

Yet, is this adequate? Many have argued that it cannot be that the only request we really make here is the request to die. It is a paradox for patient advocates to find that the grounding for this request in more and more cases has shifted, and what was called "the Resistance" emerged, in part driven by the unspoken questions of the case of Mr. C: Had we really done enough? Had we erred? In response came the disabilities rights movement, turning from civil rights and access to the larger question of meaning. The radical group "Not Dead Yet" took on the cause of treatment withdrawal and, by the end of the Schiavo case, was poised to oppose it fiercely. Death, for them, represented nothing less then abandonment.

And thus we came to the crossroads of the other video, the Schiavo case. Now seen years later, the two video representations form the grounds for the debate—the disability movement and the right-to-life movement accuse the hospice movement and the very structure of surrogacy of being murderous, callous, and dangerous.

Back to the Future

Moral philosophy leads us back to our question of life and its worth. Yet such cases remind us that our theory will be played out in complex ways, in the chaos of accidents and the lacuna in families, and, at the end of the day, practical issues really do need far more serious and detailed attention from our field. (As philosopher Emmanuel Levinas reminds us, "Even if you think that death and time are merely ectasia, the philosopher still needs to go out and buy a watch.")

Moral status is largely a religious matter, but in the final analysis, all the state can do is criminalize or permit behavior, not adjudicate belief. Each family will still need to decide the path and fate of the people they love. The criteria by which we discern death, PVS, and minimally conscious states, how we understand and study what consciousness is—and what love demands—are surely different sorts of questions. And each differs as well from the public questions: What resources, held in common, will support this moral appeal or that one, when death is a public act, health care funded or not, the gaze attentive to the family or not?

What links the two cases? In some way, the lessons of particularity and odd privileging of the debate in the case of Mrs. Schiavo needs to be understood in light of our shared culture anxieties. It ought to be noted by any religious ethicist that without universal access to health care, well-staffed hospitals and hospices with well-trained nurses, the question of "treatment withdrawal" will be framed entirely economically. The budget for motorized wheelchairs was cut from federal Medicaid funding because, explained the administration, recipients "were scamming" the system. Had Mrs. Schiavo not had her feeding tube withdrawn, she would have faced the most significant relative cuts in state and federal funding since the program began. Research funding for all basic and translational research was significantly reduced a year after this case. An unfinished task of health care reform is this issue of resource allocation, and the problem of worth cannot be de-contextualized from the tragic limits of care faced by most families. We have insisted and taught that families need to understand that medicine cannot always cure, yet our ethical reflections need to include texts about debt and social limits and about what is a public and what a private cost, which in the classic and religious textual tradition was always a central debate. In this way, what the case of Mrs. Schiavo lacked was this aspect of religious reflection, as opposed to too much religious reflection, as was commonly assumed.

Two Categories of Things

Brain death criteria and the first literature about PVS were attempts to draw a bright line across a murky biological issue—to solve with biological criteria that larger and complex moral problem that is the task of faith communities throughout human history, for death and its borders is also a matter of faith and its commitments. It is no surprise that the line will keep shifting, not a failure to note that MRIs give more and different data, or that new criteria are still needed.

It is critical to understand that the line was always an attempt to relate two separate categories of things—moral events and physical events—and cross-category relationships are always imperfect. In this way, this chapter itself is a crossing of borders in the uncertain darkness of an unfinished field, a night crossing that resists the clarity of easy claim, easy cases, and known terrain—for in asking for reflection of faith communities on the story of Mrs. Schiavo, I have instead given you another story, another video, and it has not helped to make the case clearly; it has added another complexity. Hence, it is a manifestation of how casuistry, the Talmudic method, the Sharia texts of Islam, or the stories of the Buddha work.

A person is a bag of stories, and we take them out, and we exchange them. Every American, indeed every person in reach of the flickering light of CNN on this globe, will die with the memory of the tape of Mrs. Schiavo as an image—as you read these words, you can picture the mother, the daughter, the balloon, the lace at the collar of the nightgown. I have added a second story and you, reader and I, teller, will die with his story in us, so it is important that we understand it fully (for it is all that is left of him); that we understand why and how we might have failed or succeeded in both of these cases. Each person, like our cases, is a story that faces us and then enters and lives in us. We are, in the account of Emmanuel Levinas, interrupted by the question of the other, who comes to us with her naked, still face, and his vulnerable eyes, who interrupts our monologue about grand ideas in bioethics because we then must stop and respond to her problem, because her life depends on us. Even the grace of death will depend on us in modernity.

Usually cases like the "easy" one on the videotape are never seen by committees anymore—if everyone agrees, why even listen? We in bioethics, like the media, only appear in Big Trouble: We make our theology and our bioethics about the large public tragedies of the Schiavo family, we teach about extremes. But this is an error, for most families struggle in far more ordinary ways, making the sort of choices we construct by theories made at the margins, in cases where the choices seem far more defined—hence my bringing of the alternate case against The Case, and I would ask you, reader, to think of them together, to think complexly about the sort of question that is being asked of us by this sort of death.

Is normativity possible in such a chapter as this one, or must we only agree to a naturalistic and descriptive account of religious ethics, noting at least the passion of all sides in the debate and their obvious love and sincerity? In this, I would argue that an American answer is still possible: In case of religious dissent, the state must allow the greatest measure of individual freedom, and this is expressed in families, when individuals falter, because we trust that one's family will love you uniquely and finally.

Religious responses to the Schiavo case varied widely, even within the Catholic moral tradition, and generalizing about faith responses will not give an accurate picture of the task of the scholar of religion and ethics. Such a task is better met by the narrative multivocality I have modeled here, one that asks not after our rights, but our fundamental duties at the end of life. Here I would suggest a core duty is to receive the narratives of faith in their particularity, yet to understand their incommensurability. Yet, in a world of incommensurate claims, we have a duty even when we have no other, and that is to listen to despair without despairing, and to question even that thing we think is most true—that such cases are easy.

NOTES TO CHAPTER 7

1. This point could be assessed in a small, empirical study: One could ask after the speaker's fees of prominent bioethicists and discern what percentage derived from the various "hot topics in bioethics," notably the Schiavo case, and ironically, "conflicts of interests" . . . then use a control, say, "poor children," to understand and track this phenomenon.
2. Philosopher Sam Flieshacker points out that when a moral philosopher says she is working on this topic, laypeople say impatiently, "Golly, haven't you guys figured that one out yet?" See Flieshacker, S. What does

it mean to say a life is worth living? Paper delivered at Northwestern University Philosophy Seminar Series, Evanston, IL, Fall 2005.

3. Belling, C. The night of the living dead. Paper at Northwestern University, Evanston, IL, Spring 2006. In this work, Belling notes that it was the doctors' contention in the Quinlan case that "family members had no right to decisions about treatment withdrawal."

4. Cf. "We Love Our Tubes" from the Not Dead Yet website: http://www. notdeadyet.org/docs/weloveourtubes032605.html.

5. Zoloth, L., and Sieden, D.J. Really, really dead. Paper and response, Kaiser Foundation annual meeting, 1988, and Summer Bioethics Seminar, 1990.

6. Whose name and that of the children were not published for fear of reprisal.

7. Eck, D.L. *A New Religious America: How a "Christian Country" Has Become the World's Most Religiously Diverse Nation.* San Francisco: HarperCollins, 2002. In this work, as in the Harvard Project on New Religions, Eck clearly demonstrates the mainstreaming of Islam, Bahá'í, Buddhism, and Hinduism in urban and suburban communities.

8. Stuart Sarbacker, personal communication, May 2005.

9. Les Friedman, personal communication, May 2005.

10. Amundsen, D.W. The medieval Catholic tradition. In R.L. Numbers and D.W. Amundsen, eds. *Caring and Curing: Health and Medicine in the Western Religious Traditions.* New York: Macmillan, 1986, pp. 65–107.

11. McCormick, R.A. Physician-assisted suicide: Flight from compassion. *Christian Century* 1991;108(35):1132–1143.

12. Bresnehan, J.F. Catholic spirituality and medical interventions in dying. *America* 1991;164(14):670–675.

13. Ibid.

14. Hurwitz, P.J., Picard, J. and Steinberg, A., eds. *Jewish Ethics and the Care of End-of-Life Patients: A Collection of Rabbinical, Bioethical, Philosophical, and Juristic Opinions.* Jersey City, NJ: KTAV, 2006. Cf. Steinberg, A. The Steinberg commission for the treatment of the terminally ill patient. *Assia* 2002;69–70:5–58. Also, Vardit Ravitsky makes the case for the permissibility of withdrawal under these circumstances, while noting that other consideration are at stake for nutrition and hydration: Ravitsky, V. Timers on ventilators. *British Medical Journal* 2005;330:415–417.

15. Fletcher, J. Clinical ethics. Society for Bioethics Consultation, St. Louis, September 1990.

16. Allison, D. Compassion. In Mosley, W. and Kenison, K., eds. *The Best American Short Stories 2003: Selected from U.S. and Canadian Magazines.* Boston: Houghton Mifflin Harcourt, 2003, pp. 318–319.

17. Ibid., p. 298.

18. Ibid., p. 320.

19. Ibid., pp. 322–323.

8 ::

Disability Rights and Wrongs in the Terri Schiavo Case

Lawrence J. Nelson

Although the struggle over the fate of Terri Schiavo was waged in Florida and federal courts and in the media primarily by her husband and her parents, many other individuals and organizations enthusiastically and loudly joined in as well, including proponents of a right to die, health care workers, religious fundamentalists, politicians, right-to-life proponents, opponents of euthanasia and assisted suicide, lawyers, bioethicists—and disability rights activists. On October 15, 2003, Ms. Schiavo's gastrostomy tube was removed for the second time pursuant to a court order. On October 21, the Florida Legislature passed "Terri's Law," which authorized the governor to issue an executive order directing the reinsertion of the tube. Governor Jeb Bush signed the bill and issued the order. On that same day, Michael Schiavo, her husband, filed a lawsuit arguing that "Terri's Law" was unconstitutional and seeking an injunction to stop reinsertion of the tube; but the tube was reinserted anyway, and the controversy continued.

On October 23, 2003, just two days after "Terri's Law" changed her fate again, 23 national disability organizations publicly issued a statement "in support of Terri Schindler-Schiavo, and her human and civil rights" that opposed stopping use of her gastrostomy tube for the provision of nutrition and hydration. They described themselves as "the national spokespersons for the rights of millions of Americans with disabilities whose voices are often not heard over the din of political and religious rhetoric."[1] The driving force behind these organizations' opposition to the discontinuance of Ms. Schiavo's nutrition and hydration was their conclusion that this action violated her rights and the rights of disabled people generally. They argued that Ms. Schiavo "deserves nothing less than the full advantage of human and civil rights the rest of us are fortunate to enjoy as Americans. . . . [T]he life-and-death issues surrounding [Ms. Schiavo] are first and foremost disability rights issues—issues which affect millions of Americans with disabilities, old and young."[2]

Curiously, despite their assertion that the case is "first and foremost" about rights, the organizations never specified which rights of Ms. Schiavo—and of the disabled generally—would be violated by removing her gastrostomy tube, an action that would lead to her death. Nevertheless, I interpret the text of this statement, as well as the related claims made by other commentators on disability, as making clear that one basic right is at the core of their concern: the right of persons not to suffer disadvantage because the group (whether natural or artificial) to which they belong is the object of prejudice, contempt, or wrongful discrimination.[3] Put differently, no one should suffer because he or she is a member of a group thought less worthy of respect, as a group, than others. This right truly does belong to all, disabled or not.

In my view, two core convictions about disability drive the disability rights advocates' (DRAs) reaction in the case of Terri Schiavo. First, disabled persons are consistently made the targets of profound prejudice by the "normal" population, including the family members of disabled persons. The members of this population explicitly or implicitly participate in what has been called the "ideology of normalcy," which routinely devalues and dismisses the disabled. The DRAs were convinced that Ms. Schiavo was the object of prejudice because she was disabled when her husband and the Florida courts decided to remove her gastrostomy tube and allow her to die. In other words, the DRAs perceived the cessation of Ms. Schiavo's life-sustaining treatment in itself as an insult to disabled people because it was generated by and signaled contempt for the disabled.

Second, whatever happens to one disabled person directly affects all disabled people. The mistreatment of one disabled person threatens all disabled people with mistreatment. This is akin to the feminist conviction that "the personal is political": whatever happens to one woman, because she is a woman, affects all women. Whatever happens to one disabled person, because she is disabled, affects all disabled people. This fear of a slippery slope was behind the DRAs' position in the Schiavo case: If her feeding tube can be removed, then tube feeding can be denied to any disabled person. To avoid this terrible outcome, they must oppose forgoing use of her feeding tube. The DRAs were also concerned that terminating Ms. Schiavo's treatment was based on the notion that different, less exacting ethical and legal standards apply to the disabled than to the able-bodied.

The DRAs' two core convictions directly led them, indeed drove them, to adopt certain ethical and legal positions and to advance certain types of arguments in Terri Schiavo's case (and others as well) because she is a disabled person. Part I of this chapter delves into some foundational questions. What does it mean to be disabled? How do the DRAs understand disability? Was Terri Schiavo disabled, and why does it matter?

To illuminate the meaning and significance of disability for the DRAs and how they used it in the Schiavo case, I will present Tom Koch's distinction between the "ideology of normalcy," which he claims is adopted and utilized by "contemporary medicine and mainline bioethics," and the "ideology of difference,"[4] which he endorses. Koch calls both positions "ideologies" because they possess a certain set of moral, social, and political values; he perceives them as expressing "two different concepts of humanness and the nature of persons within a society" as well.[5]

My view is that the essence, the hard center, of Koch's "ideology of normalcy" has been adopted and used by that group of people and organizations I call the DRAs who were opposed to discontinuance of Ms. Schiavo's gastrostomy tube for nutrition and hydration. I acknowledge that not all persons and organizations who hold themselves out as DRAs will hold to this ideology in precisely the way Koch describes it and that they are not necessarily all acting in deliberate concert. Nevertheless, I find their core beliefs close enough to characterize them fairly as more or less axiologically integrated in this manner, and I hope my exposition will adequately justify my admittedly rough characterization of the views on disability and the rights of the disabled of these separate organizations and individuals.

Part II will discuss how the DRAs' convictions lead them either to perceive facts differently when a question of forgoing life-sustaining medical treatment (LST) for a disabled person has arisen or to ignore, distort, or twist the facts—and the law—to suit their ends. I conclude that no one should distort or ignore factual evidence or fail to give facts proper attention, as the DRAs did in the Schiavo case, in order to advance some strategic or ideological goal. Part III will explore how in order to protect the disabled from prejudice, the DRAs vehemently argue that: (1) The clear and convincing evidence test is the only one that should be used to determine when LST may be forgone; (2) surrogates, whether family members, judges, or other strangers, cannot be trusted to make correct decisions about LST for the disabled; and (3) even mentally competent disabled adults ought not to be permitted to refuse LST. I shall argue that all of these positions are deeply flawed.

⠅⠅ Part I: The Meaning and Significance of Disability

The DRAs on Disability

According to Koch, the ideology of difference—which he and other DRAs embrace—assumes that all individuals are "incomplete and unable" and holds that disability "is not an inherent limit but an outcome resulting from society's rejection of a person on the basis of his or her difference—its devaluing of his or her status, which endangers both social function and existential worth." The difference in the disabled is therefore "not necessarily disabling." Disability is instead an outcome rooted in "discriminatory social reaction to the effects of this or that difference." Disabilities, then, are really just differences or neutral forms of variation in people's physical or cognitive function that are "not necessarily disabling" and do not pose any "inherent limit" on the individual.[6] Disabilities are not a set of medical problems, but the outcomes of invidious social discrimination and prejudice.

In contrast, the ideology of normalcy sees an individual who has any loss of cognitive, physical, or sensory ability when compared to the normal population as having a "disability" (a pathological condition that ought to be handled by the medical profession) and as being "necessarily disadvantaged" thereby. These deviations or differences from the norm are "by definition, a harm resulting in suffering to be avoided where possible," and a person having such differences is "by definition . . . limited, his or her status unnatural." If a difference is "sufficiently severe, the person is assumed [by one holding the ideology of normalcy] to be diminished, lessened both existentially and as a member of the social constituency that we share. . . . In the extreme, severe deviations from the norm result in a life unworthy of continuance, one so devalued as to be disqualified from . . . the 'sanctity of [human] life.'" Closely connected to severe disability when "the harm [is] extensive" is "the assumption . . . that death is necessarily preferable—more natural than continued existence." At a minimum, to be "disabled is to have a lesser endowment, to be unable to experience the world in a way similar to that of other . . . individuals" who are assumed to be "discrete, self-reliant, self-conscious" persons. A disabled person "by definition is limited, his or her status unnatural." Because a disabled individual is diminished and unnatural,

> termination [of life] becomes a rational response to chronically limited ability, a logical action ending or preventing the suffering that accompanies the harm that necessarily accrues to the person . . . whose social posture [is] severely limited by restrictions imposed by a disability.

Koch sees both "contemporary medicine and mainline bioethics" as embracing the ideology of normalcy.[7]

In my interpretation of Koch, the ideology of normalcy can be summarized by three basic propositions: (1) All disabilities are bad, undesirable, pathological conditions; (2) all disabled persons are necessarily disadvantaged by their disabilities and suffer a decreased quality of life; and (3) all disabled people are morally disvalued, diminished, and discriminated against because they are disabled; furthermore, they are by and large considered expendable; they can be killed or allowed to die at will, they can be eliminated.

Other DRAs use some different terms to identify the same phenomenon, but they also affirm Koch's basic claims about disability being bad, the disabled being seriously disadvantaged, and the discrimination and devaluation faced by the disabled. Amundson and Taira call the phenomenon "ableism."

> Bodily differences are not the causes of [the] problems [of the disabled], a destructive social prejudice is to blame; we call it ableism. Ableism is a doctrine that falsely treats impairments as inherently and naturally horrible and blames the impairments themselves for the problems experienced by the people who have them. Ableism is wrong. Disability is a social problem, not a medical problem. Impairments are not the problem; ableism is.[8]

Saxton calls this phenomenon the "medical system's view" of disability and points out its "fundamental assumption . . . that greater degrees of disability (defined by medical standards as increased pathology) are associated with decreased quality of life."[9] The 23 organizations that issued the Schiavo statement affirmed the devaluation experienced by the disabled: "People with severe cognitive disabilities are devalued as lives not worth living. In truth, *the lives of all of us with severe disabilities* are often considered expendable."[10] Bickenbach calls the "social devaluation of the life of persons with disabilities, as a matter of both attitude and practice" a "fact" and describes our world as one "in which physical and mental disability [are] systematically viewed as ground for judging a life to be of less value, or indeed of no value at all."[11] Coleman and Gill state that "disability-based discrimination in this culture is deep-seated, virtually unconscious, pervasive and overwhelming."[12]

Another Perspective on the Meaning of "Disability"
Before considering how the DRAs' views on disability relate to the Schiavo case, let's first consider a different framework for understanding the meaning of "disability." The World Health Organization has distinguished impairment, disability, and handicap in a manner useful to this discussion:

> An impairment is an abnormality or loss of any physiological or anatomical structure, or function. Disability refers to the consequences of an impairment, that is, any restriction or loss of ability to perform an activity in the manner or within the range considered appropriate for nonimpaired persons. Handicap is the social disadvantage that results from an impairment or a disability.[13]

In this framework, a disability flows from an impairment and is a restriction on or loss of an ability to perform an activity typically appropriate for persons who lack the abnormal physiological or anatomical structure. A handicap is the discrimination or prejudice inflicted on disabled persons (the "social disadvantage") as "a result of social choices; they are not part of the 'fabric of the universe.' Because they are chosen, they can be changed."[14] Applying this framework, it cannot be doubted that Ms. Schiavo had impairments (i.e., abnormalities or losses of physiological or anatomical structures or functions). Plainly, the most significant and serious abnormality of an anatomical structure that she had was the damage done to her brain by a cardiac arrest. The autopsy showed that her brain was "grossly abnormal and weighed only 615 grams (1.35 lbs)," less than half of the expected weight for an adult of her age.[15] This is a very significant finding because brain weight "is an important index of its pathologic state."[16] Interestingly, the 645 mL of cerebrospinal fluid recovered upon opening her skull weighed 63 grams more than her brain.[17] In sum, her cerebral cortex was badly damaged by hypoxic-ischemic encephalopathy as a result of the cardiac arrest she suffered. Yet her brain stem was relatively intact, as was demonstrated by her ability to breathe on her own, to have sleep–wake cycles, and to demonstrate reflex actions mediated by the brain stem. At the time of her death, at least, she had several other impairments as well: extreme muscle atrophy, severe osteoporosis, urolithiasis (kidney stones), heterotopic ossification (abnormal formation of true bone within extraskeletal soft tissue), degenerative joint changes, glossal, pharyngeal, and neck muscle atrophy, and an inability to swallow.[18]

Ms. Schiavo also had a "disability" as the term is used by WHO: the massive cortical brain damage she suffered as a result of the cardiac arrest had the consequence of rendering her completely unconscious (she was in a permanent vegetative state, sometimes—albeit inaccurately in this case—called persistent vegetative state[19]). This clinical diagnosis of permanent vegetative state was confirmed by CT scans that "demonstrated massive atrophy of the cerebral hemispheres, indicating irreversibility (permanency) of the patient's clinical condition, and the EEG's showed no cerebral activity, confirming the fact that the patient was unconscious and unaware (vegetative state)."[20] In other words, it could be said that she had the *ultimate* disability (putting aside death itself): she lost the ability to engage in *any* conscious or deliberate activity *at all*; she could not experience *anything*, think *anything*, feel *anything*, or move *any* part of her body voluntarily.

However, application of the WHO understanding of "disability" to Ms. Schiavo (and all others like her) is highly problematic conceptually. Application of the common meaning of disability—"a disadvantage or deficiency, especially a physical or mental impairment that interferes with or prevents normal achievement in a particular area"—to this case is likewise deeply problematic.[21] The difficulty here was ably pointed out by a group of Florida bioethicists commenting upon political developments after Ms. Schiavo's death:

> [I]t is widely and accurately agreed that a person who is permanently unconscious is most certainly not disabled in either the ordinary or the medical use of the term. To be disabled is to be in some way physiologically harmed or different such that the patient is unable in varying degrees to do or experience things that other people do or experience. If someone is unable to do or experience *anything*, it is incoherent to suggest that such a person is *disabled* in the sense of having less-than-customary capacity. To be permanently unconscious is not to have limitations, impediments or decreased functions. These properties, however, are precisely and exclusively required to define disability; without these characteristics, one is not disabled.[22]

Ms. Schiavo did not have a loss of ability to perform a normal activity or set of normal activities; she did not have a physical or mental impairment that interfered with normal achievement in a particular area of life. She lost her entire ability to experience herself and her world in any manner. She was alive biologically, but she no longer had *a* life. "One's *life* . . . is immensely important; it is the sum of one's aspirations, decisions, activities, projects, and human relationships."[23]

Severely physically disabled adults have a personal, biographical life. Like everyone else, they have aspirations, plans, hopes, and human relationships. Their physical impairments shape these plans and relationships to some extent or another, but do not eliminate them. Severely mentally disabled adults retain some ability to experience themselves and their environment (including other persons) and to interact with their environment and the people in it. They too have a personal, biographical life, although its breadth and complexity will be circumscribed.

However, Ms. Schiavo's severe and irreversible brain damage put her beyond disability, beyond suffering physiological or anatomical impairment of function, beyond a decreased ability to engage in typical activities and to have commonly encountered experiences. She no longer could have any aspirations, make any decisions, engage in any activities or projects, have any human relationships of which she was aware. Others could relate to her, but she was unable to relate with them or to manifest her own character, values, and preferences to them. Consequently, Terri Schiavo was not disabled because she had lost *all* ability to have any kind of a biographical, personal life. Her permanently unconscious state does not make her a moral or legal nonperson, an object, but it does rob her of all purposeful mental and physical function in the world and radically transforms her.

Was Ms. Schiavo "handicapped" in the meaning given by WHO— that is, was she socially disadvantaged or discriminated against as a result of her massive brain damage? When her husband Michael sought to have her gastrostomy tube removed so that she would be allowed to die in accordance with what he understood her wishes to have been, and when the Florida courts made the decision on her behalf to refuse further use of the tube, was she morally and legally wronged as a result of bias against the disabled? Here is the critical ethical issue; here is where the meaning of "disability" according to the DRAs generates its most direct and serious implications; and here is where the significance of the disagreement about whether Terri Schiavo was disabled or not ultimately resides.

The DRA Position on the Schiavo Case

Koch's ideology of difference characterizes "disability" as an outcome of society's invidiously discriminatory reaction to the effects of a person's physical or mental difference, not as an "inherent limit." From this perspective, difference is created by the social devaluation of the disabled person, not by variations in physical or mental function. Consequently, Ms. Schiavo had no "inherent limit" placed on her by her severe brain damage, nor was she disabled by this damage, but she was disabled by the reaction of society to her difference—a reaction that made her expendable.

Furthermore, the DRAs categorized Ms. Schiavo as "disabled" in *their* understanding due to both the application of the ideology of normalcy to her and their own core convictions. Accordingly, her brain damage was considered a bad, pathological condition just like all disabilities. As a disabled person and like all other disabled persons, Ms. Schiavo necessarily was disadvantaged and had a decreased quality of life. But most importantly to the DRAs, because she was disabled and had a bad quality of life, she was necessarily disvalued and diminished, she was expendable, killable—just like all other persons with disabilities. And this is exactly the way she was treated by her husband, the Florida court system, and all those who supported removing the tube—as someone who had no rights, no value. As the DRAs see it, when all of these individuals sought her death by removing the tube, they engaged in invidious discrimination against the handicapped.

The two core convictions of the DRAs (as described above) drove their response to the Schiavo case. First, they perceived Ms. Schiavo as just one more disabled person who was the target of prejudice by the normal population who routinely devalue and dismiss the disabled. The DRAs saw here the application by the physicians, judges, and those who supported her husband of "the premise that death is better than disability."[24] "We know that life with a disability is worth living, and we know what makes life awful for us is the attitude of 'better off dead' that drives much of the thinking surrounding people like Terri Schindler-Schiavo."[25] The depth of the DRAs' convictions about the deadly nature and intent of those who apply the ideology of normalcy to the disabled can be seen in these words of Diane Coleman:

> The medical profession generally devalues people with disabilities. Doctors too often induce families to give up on the severely disabled. The bioethicists in particular have warped the end-of-life care movement into a life-ending movement. They want to be able to kill behind the closed doors of a room in a hospital or nursing home.[26]

The second core conviction of the DRAs was heavily in play in the Schiavo case as well, the conviction that whatever happens to one disabled person directly affects all disabled people. The DRAs who issued the statement in opposition to removing Ms. Schiavo's tube—and, to use their words, "in support of Terri Schindler-Schiavo"—clearly perceived this case as essentially linked to all disabled people. They described their statement as telling "the real story about Terri Schindler-Schiavo, *and thousands like her.*" They described the "life-and-death issues" of the Schiavo case as *"first and foremost* disability rights issues—issues *which affect millions* of Americans with disabilities, old and young." They argued the inherent dangerousness of the "belief that people with disabilities like [Ms. Schiavo's] are 'better off dead' is longstanding but wrong. *It imperils us all.*" They strongly asserted that they will "not rest until her most basic humanity is secure" because they believe that Ms. Schiavo loses her basic humanity by being labeled "disabled," meaning bad, undignified, expendable, worthy of death.[27] Consequently, they must oppose this conceptualization of disability and the actions based upon it for their own good, for their own survival.

The DRAs' position on the meaning and significance of disability generally and on the Schiavo case in particular is quite problematic for several reasons, although they make some telling points as well. First, contrary to the views of the DRAs (or at least their rhetoric), the disabled are by no means all alike; they do not truly constitute a uniform, thoroughly similarly situated class of persons. The range of impairments that can be called "disabilities" is staggering—from an otherwise "normal" 12-year-old with a slightly deformed leg who cannot run well, to a young adult with a cognitive impairment who works in the community and takes care of herself but needs to live in a group home, to an elderly person with advanced Alzheimer's who recognizes no one and can no longer speak intelligibly (and much in between). To be sure, all of them may be subject to invidiously discriminatory treatment in one form or another—and of course such behavior is unethical and should never be tolerated—but their status as "disabled" alone does not make them identical for any purpose, including when questions about forgoing life-sustaining medical treatment arise. It is not realistic or fair to regard "all disabilities as a generic class and treat[. . .] them as if equal."[28]

Second, the position of the DRAs, that disability is not about impairment at all but really about the negative reactions of nondisabled persons to those who have a physical or mental impairment, is too narrow. Non-trivial impairments and disabilities do, to one extent or another, alter an individual's possible projects, prospects, and opportunities—although there is no doubt that these are too heavily influenced by our society's lamentable failure to meet the needs of the disabled and to provide them much better access to personal assistance services. Therefore, the view of some DRAs who "hold that the only drawbacks of disability result from prejudice and discrimination, and that, inherently, 'it is . . . good to be disabled'"[29] is extreme and inaccurate. It is emphatically *not* good to be, like Ms. Schiavo, permanently unconscious. Nor is it inherently good and desirable to have any serious disability, although it is simultaneously true that any disability will almost surely seem worse to the able-bodied and will not uncommonly be made much worse by society's failure to change its attitudes about disability and to ameliorate the effects of impairment.

Similarly, the DRAs' view, described above, that all impairments and disabilities are neutral or merely forms of variation, isn't plausible, even though their likely reason for advancing this position is, unfortunately, only too credible: "to counter all-too-prevalent stereotypical thinking about disability as inherently bad, inherently disadvantageous, inherently a problem."[30] Steinbock urges that a distinction be made between a disability being a disadvantage and its being disadvantageous on balance, and asks us to consider the example of the brilliant violinist, Itzhak Perlman. He walks slowly with braces and canes due to polio as a child, and this is "certainly a disadvantage [and probably one he would prefer not to have]. But is Perlman disadvantaged on balance due to his disability? Surely not; we should all be so disadvantaged."[31] Yet if someone intentionally injected a substance into someone's legs for the purpose of taking away his ability to walk easily and forcing him to walk as Mr. Perlman must, we would surely consider the agent to have committed a serious moral and legal wrong against both the now-disabled person and society.[32]

Impairments and disabilities can be, though not *necessarily* are, problems or limitations of one kind or another for the person who has them; it certainly depends on their nature and seriousness and on the particular perspective of the individual person. One disability rights advocate has acknowledged this: "Not all problems of disability are socially created and, thus, theoretically remediable. . . . The inability to move without mechanical aid, to see, to hear, or to learn is not inherently neutral. Disability itself limits some options."[33] Moreover, different people will react to the limitations imposed upon them by disability in different ways: One size of response to disability does not fit all.

Third, although it is obvious that the DRAs are convinced that many people, both "normal" and disabled,[34] accept the "the premise that death is better than disability," anyone who does is at the very least foolish and ill-informed—and probably morally obtuse and prejudiced (in the literal sense of judging something too soon) about disability as well. The same applies to those able-bodied individuals who were part of a telephone survey in Oregon and who "surmised . . . that if they were confined to a wheelchair, they would rather be dead."[35] "The able-bodied fail to appreciate how much they would enjoy their life if they acquired an impairment."[36]

Many of us have some kind of impairment now, and almost all of us will have some significant physical or cognitive impairment before we die. We are all dependent on others to one extent or another for help in living now, and unless we die suddenly, we are very likely to be dependent on others for assistance as we age and approach the end of our lives. Therefore, I join Amundson and Taira (and other DRAs) in rejecting the values and attitudes embraced by those who say, "Wouldn't you rather die than have someone else wipe your butt?"[37] or "Wouldn't you rather be dead than disabled?"

Nevertheless, this is not to say that I don't care about my ability to take care of my own personal hygiene or about being significantly disabled for the remainder of my life: I would much rather handle such matters on my own and not be disabled. But it is utterly wrong and presumptive to claim that having these preferences, however strongly they are held, means that I also am biased against such persons and believe that those who need this form of personal assistance from others are lesser human beings or should kill themselves—or be killed—in order to be rid of them. It is neither necessarily irrational nor an expression of ugly, mindless prejudice against the disabled for an individual to conscientiously choose not to continue living due to the burdensomeness of her existence to herself, or due to her desire to avoid certain consequences for her loved ones if she remained alive. This can also be true for a surrogate (such as a parent of a developmentally disabled child) to make a decision about forgoing life-sustaining treatment for a child who cannot choose for himself. I discuss these points further in Part III below.

Finally, I am not sure quite what to make of Coleman's empirical claim that physicians generally devalue people with disabilities and too often induce families to "give up on the severely disabled" and, I presume, let them die wrongfully. (The antipathy and distrust of the

DRAs toward the medical profession has been often noted.[38]) Disabled people (not to mention the poor, the uninsured, the homeless, the chronically mentally ill, drug abusers, women, people of color, illegal aliens, and so on) surely do receive inferior health care too often, and prejudice probably plays a large role here. Undoubtedly, this should be morally condemned. But this does not mean that it is wrong to forgo medical treatment in any individual case involving a disabled person. Coleman's sweeping claim that bioethicists want to "kill [the disabled and others] behind the closed doors of a room in a hospital or nursing home" is bizarre, unsupported by evidence (other than references to Peter Singer's writings), and irresponsible, although she is not the only DRA to make it.[39]

:: Part II: Facts, Evidence, and Values

The core convictions of the DRAs led them to perceive and interpret certain key facts about the Schiavo case in a certain manner. Specifically, they outright denied that Ms. Schiavo was in the permanent vegetative state, or at least tried to cast serious doubt upon the validity of this diagnosis and prognosis. They also flatly asserted that she had been denied rehabilitative services by her husband. In my view, however one characterizes what they did in these two regards (ignoring, distorting, spinning, twisting, or merely interpreting the facts), they can be understood to have used—manipulated, actually—the "facts and evidence" in order to better achieve their end of protecting the disabled from medicine's, bioethics', and society's prejudice or spite. In other words, by portraying Ms. Schiavo as conscious and treatable in fact and by asserting as fact that she was denied rehabilitation services, the DRAs could ground their claim that she was the victim of invidious discrimination against the disabled. A detailed examination of both these factual issues follows.

Most notably, the DRAs—along with many other partisans—denied that Ms. Schiavo was in a permanent vegetative state. They observe that Ms. Schiavo "is said to be in a 'persistent vegetative state.' But is she? In court, the medical experts were divided."[40] The *amicus curiae* brief of a variety of disability rights organizations urging reversal of Florida Judge George Greer's order denying the Schindlers' motion for relief from judgment noted that two medical experts who testified at the evidentiary hearing in 2002 "found Ms. Schiavo was not in a persistent vegetative state and that certain untried therapies would give Ms. Schiavo a good chance of recovery." Similarly, they asserted, "Despite hearing evidence from doctors with 'very impressive credentials' that Ms. Schiavo was not in a persistent vegetative state, and despite finding that she exhibited signs of cognition and thought, the court authorized her death,"[41] which makes it seem as if the judge ignored solid evidence in order to justify her death. They also claimed, "It is clear that she is conscious and responsive beyond mere reflexes, as has been demonstrated by her ability to track with her eyes, respond to verbal commands by physicians who examined her on video, and react to those she loves."[42] Diane Coleman, President of Not Dead Yet (one of the most active of the disability rights organizations), stated that "Terri wasn't really in PVS. . . ."[43] The *amicus* brief of the International Task Force on the denial of the motion for relief from judgment asserts that:

> Since the video recordings which have been submitted to this Court clearly indicate that Terri responds and interacts with others, she does not fit within Florida's definition of PVS. . . . After objectively viewing the video-recordings of Terri, no one can reasonably claim that she is unconscious. No one can reasonably believe that she experiences nothing. The evidence clearly indicates her responsiveness.[44]

What is the evidence that Ms. Schiavo was permanently unconscious? In his order of February 11, 2000, after the initial hearing on Michael Schiavo's petition for the court to authorize the removal of her gastrostomy tube based on her wishes, Judge Greer found:

> beyond all doubt that [Ms. Schiavo] is in a persistent vegetative state . . . per the specific testimony of Dr. James Barnhill and corroborated by Dr. Vincent Gambone. The medical evidence before this court conclusively establishes that she has no hope of ever regaining consciousness and therefore capacity. . . . The film offered into evidence by [the Schindlers] does nothing to change these medical opinions which are supported by the CAT scans in evidence. Mrs. Schindler has testified as her perceptions [sic] regarding her daughter and the court is not unmindful that *perceptions may become reality to the person having them*. But the overwhelming credible evidence is that Terri Schiavo has been totally unresponsive since lapsing into the coma almost ten years ago, that her movements are reflexive and predicated on brain stem activity alone, that she suffers from severe structural brain damage and to a large extent her brain has been replaced by spinal fluid, that with the exception of one witness whom the court finds to be so biased as to lack credibility, her movements are occasional and totally consistent with the testimony of the expert medical witnesses.[45]

Given the uncontradicted medical evidence about her condition (and the Schindlers would have had the opportunity to contradict it) and the lack of any credible evidence to the contrary, Judge Greer drew the only conclusion he could: Ms. Schiavo was unconscious and would remain so. The three-judge appellate panel that later reviewed Judge Greer's conclusion about her medical condition independently concurred with it and found much more than substantial evidence[46] to support it:

> The evidence is *overwhelming* that Theresa is in a permanent or persistent vegetative state. It is important to understand that a persistent vegetative state is not simply a coma. She is not asleep. She has cycles of apparent wakefulness and apparent sleep without any cognition or awareness. As she breathes, she often makes moaning sounds. . . . Over the span of this last decade, Theresa's brain has deteriorated because of the lack of oxygen it suffered at the time of the heart attack. By mid-1996, the CAT scans of her brain showed a severely abnormal structure. *At this point, much of her cerebral cortex is simply gone and has been replaced by cerebral spinal fluid. Medicine cannot cure this condition.* Unless an act of God, a true miracle, were to recreate her brain, Theresa will always remain in an unconscious, reflexive state. . . .'[47]

The Schindlers continued to oppose removing her gastrostomy tube and later disputed that their daughter was permanently unconscious by claiming that she could improve with treatment. Their arguments to this effect were considered by the same appellate court some 6 months later:

> [A]t this time, the Schindlers have not seriously contested the fact that Mrs. Schiavo's brain has suffered major, permanent damage. In the initial adversary proceeding, a board-certified neurologist who had reviewed a CAT scan of Mrs. Schiavo's brain and an EEG testified that most, if not all, of Mrs. Schiavo's cerebral cortex—the portion of her brain that allows for human cognition and memory—is either totally destroyed or damaged beyond repair. . . . [T]he Schindlers have presented *no medical evidence* suggesting that any new treatment could restore to Mrs. Schiavo a level of function within the cerebral cortex that would allow her to understand her perceptions of sight and sound or to communicate or respond cognitively to those perceptions.[48]

Nevertheless, despite the lack of medical evidence that she might improve, the appellate court allowed the Schindlers to pursue a challenge to Judge Greer's order to remove the gastrostomy tube on the ground that it would no longer be equitable to enforce the order because of new circumstances. Judge Greer denied the challenge later filed by the Schindlers, and they again appealed.

In their third appeal, the Schindlers claimed that their daughter was not in a persistent vegetative state:

> What is more important, they maintain that current accepted medical treatment exists to restore her ability to eat and speak. . . . The Schindlers argue that in light of this new evidence of additional medical procedures intended to improve her condition, Mrs. Schiavo would now elect to undergo new treatment and would reverse the prior decision to withdraw life-prolonging procedures.[49]

The Schindlers submitted seven affidavits from licensed physicians who had reviewed Ms. Schiavo's medical records, considered anecdotal evidence about her condition from lay people, and viewed a brief videotape of a visit with her mother, but none of them had examined her. The Court of Appeal evaluated these affidavits as follows:

> The affidavits of the several doctors vary in content and rhetoric. Among [them], however, the most significant evidence comes from Dr. Fred Webber. Dr. Webber is an osteopathic physician . . . who claims that Mrs. Schiavo is not in a persistent vegetative state and that she exhibits "purposeful reaction to her environment. . . ." [O]nly Dr. Webber [of the seven] has gone so far as to suggest that available treatment could restore cognitive function to Mrs. Schiavo.[50]

In his statement sworn under oath, Dr. Webber claimed that he had within the past year treated patients "with brain defects similar to Mrs. Schiavo's" with a "cardiovascular medication style of therapy" and that in most cases these patients "have shown some improvement," with "improvement" meaning recovery of speech, enhanced speech clarity and complexity, release of contractures, and better awareness. He specifically stated that "based on my 26 years of practice, Mrs. Schiavo has a good opportunity to show some degree of improvement if treated with this type of therapy, although I cannot anticipate how much improvement."[51] Although the Court expressed "skepticism concerning Dr. Webber's affidavit," it nevertheless concluded it would be wrong to reject his opinion without consideration of more evidence and ordered Judge Greer to hold an evidentiary hearing on whether this new medical evidence would, in fairness to Ms. Schiavo, warrant a change in his order to remove the gastrostomy tube. The Court permitted each side to choose two physicians to examine her and evaluate her current condition, with a fifth physician, board-certified in neurology or neurosurgery who is "very experienced in the treatment of brain damage" and "independent of [the other] physicians and without any prior involvement with this family," to be chosen by Judge Greer in the event the parties couldn't agree on one (not surprisingly, they could not).[52]

Amazingly, Dr. Webber, the only physician who claimed under oath that his "cardiovascular" therapy had a good chance of possibly restoring cognitive function to Ms. Schiavo, never testified at the evidentiary hearing held in the fall of 2002 at the direction of the Court of Appeal. This physician, whose sworn testimony enabled the Schindlers to continue their legal battle, then disappeared from the litigation entirely.[53] Instead, the Schindlers offered the testimony of Drs. Maxfield and Hammesfahr, the former claiming that Ms. Schiavo could benefit from hyperbaric therapy and the latter claiming the same result from vasodilation therapy. These were the medical experts referred to by the DRAs. Judge Greer, however, found this testimony utterly unpersuasive:

> Neither Dr. Hammesfahr nor Dr. Maxfield was able to credibly testify that the treatment options they offered would significantly improve Terry Schiavo's quality of life. . . . It is clear from the evidence that these therapies are experimental insofar as the medical community is concerned with regard to patients like Terri Schiavo which is borne out by the *total absence* of supporting case studies or medical literature."[54]

While neither physician could offer any scientific data to support his claims, Judge Greer found Dr. Hammesfahr's testimony to be particularly weak:

> [W]hat undemises [sic: undermines] his creditability [sic] is that he did not present to this court any evidence other than his generalized statements as to the efficacy of his therapy on brain damaged individuals like Terry Schiavo. He testified that he has treated about 50 patients in the same or worse condition than Terry Schiavo since 1994 but he offered no names, no case studies, no videos and no tests results to support his claim that he had success in all but one of them. If his therapy is as effective as he would lead this court to believe, it is inconceivable that he would not produce clinical results of these patients he has treated. And surely the medical literature would be replete with this new, now patented, procedure. . . . Even he acknowledges that he is aware of no article or study that shows vasodilation therapy to be an effective treatment for persistent vegetative state.[55]

The other three physicians, including the independent neurologist appointed by the court,[56] all concluded that Ms. Schiavo was permanently unconscious. Ronald Cranford, a neurologist, has commented extensively on the Maxfield and Hammesfahr testimony and found it lacking any medical merit.[57]

Twenty months later, the Court of Appeals affirmed Judge Greer's ruling that Ms. Schiavo remained in a permanently unconscious state and that no treatment existed to restore her awareness. The Court observed that "the quality of evidence presented . . . was very high, and each side had ample opportunity to present detailed medical evidence. . . . It is likely that no guardianship court has ever received so much high-quality medical evidence. . . ."[58] The appellate judges, two of whom were new to the case, expressly stated that they:

> closely examined all of the evidence in this record. We have repeatedly examined the videotapes [of the physicians' exams of Ms. Schiavo], not merely watching short segments but carefully observing the tapes in their entirety. We have examined the brain scans with the eyes of educated laypersons and considered the explanations offered by the doctors. . . . We have concluded that, if we were called upon to review [Judge Greer's] decision de novo, we would still affirm it.[59]

In other words, these judges were personally persuaded that the testimony of Hammesfahr and Maxfield was nothing short of unbelievable when compared with the testimony of a number of other physicians that was supported by reliable medical studies and consistent with the clinical evidence like the CT scans showing massive atrophy of the brain and the flat EEGs showing no cortical activity.

The DRAs also claimed that Ms. Schiavo "has not undergone the rehabilitation that is typically given to people with this type [severe brain injury] of disability" in violation of "her right to therapy and support."[60] This claim, however, was not accompanied by any reference or documentation and is flatly contradicted by the facts included in the Wolfson report. Prof. Jay Wolfson was appointed Ms. Schiavo's guardian *ad litem* (GAL) pursuant to "Terri's Law"[61] and the order of the Chief Judge of Florida's 6th Judicial Circuit and produced a 38-page report sent to both Governor Bush and the chief judge who appointed him.[62] The GAL, who was previously not involved in the case and knew none of the parties, visited regularly with Ms. Schiavo, reviewed the entire court file of 13 years of litigation (including all items of evidence) as well as her clinical and medical records, interviewed the members of her family and caregivers, had discussions with medical, legal, bioethical, and religious practitioners and scholars, and conducted independent research into the substantive issues.[63]

The GAL's report documents that she received "extensive testing, therapy and observation" at Humana Northside Hospital for the first two and a half months after her cardiac arrest and thereafter was transferred to the College Park skilled care and rehabilitation facility and Bayfront Hospital, where she received "additional, aggressive rehabilitation."[64] The report also notes that she received "regular and intense physical, occupational and speech therapies," that Mr. Schiavo took her to California in the fall of 1990 for surgical placement of an experimental thalamic stimulator, and that after returning from California in January of 1991, she was transferred to Mediplex Rehabilitation Center, "where she received 24 hour skilled care, physical, occupational, speech and recreational therapies."[65] Seven months later, the GAL documented, she was transferred to another skilled care facility where "periodic neurological exams, regular and aggressive physical, occupational and speech therapy continued through 1994."[66] This evidence demonstrates that she received at the very least "typical" rehabilitation services, though probably significantly more, as shown by the experimental thalamic stimulator, a device implanted in her brain.

Immediately following the claim that Ms. Schiavo did not receive typical rehabilitation, the DRAs state that people with severe cognitive disabilities are "devalued as lives not worth living" and are "often considered expendable." This clearly implies that the absence of typical rehabilitation proves that she—and other disabled individuals—are the object of wrongful discrimination and neglect. While this may very well be true in other instances, it was not true in this case. This last point is telling: They claim things about the Schiavo case that aren't true, but which may well be true in other cases. Why do this? I see this as a tactic to tie her in with other disabled people; yet all disabled are not fundamentally alike.

However, the DRAs do make true claims as well. Here is just one:

> Historically, many people with disabilities such as autism, Down syndrome and cerebral palsy have been thought to be incapable of communication. Increasingly, yesterday's assumptions about inability are being thrown out when confronted with the reality of people exceeding the low expectations put on them by others.[67]

They are right: reality should change the minds of people who simply assume disabled people cannot function, who won't pay attention to the fact that they can communicate or otherwise act purposefully, or who habitually characterize the functioning of disabled people as insignificant. But by parity of reasoning the same point must apply to them: when they are "confronted with the reality" of a person like Ms. Schiavo who cannot communicate or perform any purposeful activity because she is permanently unconscious, they must accept it as well.

In sum, the facts and evidence carefully and repeatedly reviewed by the Florida courts (and fully confirmed by the findings of the carefully performed and extensive autopsy)[68] demonstrate that Ms. Schiavo was permanently unconscious and tragically beyond the reach of medicine's ability bring her back to consciousness. Both Judge Greer and the Court of Appeal clearly and logically explain why they arrived at their conclusions and why they found the "evidence" to the contrary to have no substance. The facts, then, do not in any way support the claims of the DRAs about her being conscious and responsive, at least when fairly considered apart from any ideological purposes that might be achieved by ignoring, editing, or spinning these facts. Why did the DRAs ignore the available facts and evidence, if not misrepresent them, and adamantly assert that she was not unconscious and could recover?

In my view, they did so in order to rescue her from unpersonhood, from the lack of moral standing and respect that they believe disability inevitably generates in the minds of the normal population. By imagining her to be conscious and responsive, the DRAs were attempting to make it obviously wrong to stop her tube feedings and deliberately to make her dead. This furthers their goal of breaking the links they believe necessarily exist between disability and lack of moral value, between disability and a low quality of life, between disability and expendability. They are trying to destroy the logic of "if she is permanently unconscious in the vegetative state, then it is clear she deserves to die, to be killed, because she's disabled." To advance their goal of protecting all disabled people from this sort of prejudice in decision making about forgoing LST, they don't look at the facts of the case fairly or objectively. Unfortunately, such distortion of the facts happens frequently in cases involving forgoing LST of disabled people.[69]

Reasonable and fair-minded people should have profound reservations about the DRAs' views when they engage in this factual gerrymandering, whether it's done purposefully or not. For one thing, it undermines the persuasiveness of the legitimate claims they advance, such as their criticism of the blind perniciousness of "better dead than disabled." Furthermore, it is wrong and dishonest for *anyone* to ignore, edit, or spin the facts of a case for ideological or strategic purposes (although lawyers seem to do this all the time—perhaps this is one of the deep problems with zealous advocacy). It would, for example, be wrong for Michael Schiavo to make his wife seem worse than she really was (i.e., to ignore or suppress legitimate evidence that she was conscious). It is likewise wrong for the DRAs or anyone else to make her condition appear better than it really is. It's nothing short of disingenuous to offer "the real story"[70] about Terri Schiavo and simultaneously pay no or selective attention to the facts and evidence.

If the facts about her medical condition as detailed above are wrong, if the DRAs, the Schindlers, or anyone else can produce reliable empirical studies that demonstrate the medical value of hyperbaric or vasodilation treatment for severely brain-damaged patients like Ms. Schiavo, then they should publicly produce that evidence. They could not do that in front of the Florida courts, which gave them every opportunity to do so (one could argue too many opportunities were offered—think of Dr. Webber's absence when he faced cross examination under oath, in front of a judge, about his extravagant medical claims). If they cannot, then no reasonable person should accept their mere assertions to the contrary or be persuaded by the misleading assertions of the DRAs that the medical experts were "divided" when some of them were making factually insupportable, indeed unbelievable, contentions about Ms. Schiavo's condition and prospects for improvement. Simply saying, even with great sincerity and conviction, that the earth is flat—or that lending money is inherently immoral—does not make either true.

:: Part III: The DRAs on Standards for Forgoing Life-Sustaining Treatment and Surrogates

When an individual is mentally incompetent to make his or her own decisions and someone raises a question about forgoing LST, the DRAs insist that LST may be forgone only if clear and convincing evidence can be produced that the individual would, under the present circumstances, refuse the treatment. In its *amicus* brief in the Schiavo case, Not Dead Yet argued that the U.S. Constitution requires use of the clear and convincing evidence standard "on a question as fundamental as life or death, because the consequences of abuse or misjudgment are both ultimate and irreversible. For this reason, neither a court nor any third party may base a decision on their own view of the affected person's 'quality of life.' Only the person's own desires may drive this determination."[71] Not Dead Yet also claimed that if reasonable minds disagree on any issue pertaining to forgoing LST, "any doubt or uncertainty counsels against death."[72] Another DRA organization made the same claims in the Wendland case, which involved a wife's attempt to stop tube feeding of her husband over the objection of the patient's estranged mother, although he, unlike Ms. Schiavo, was minimally conscious:

> [The legal and moral right to life should create] a strong presumption in favor of life . . . that might be overcome only with clear and convincing evidence that this is what the affected person would have wanted under the circumstances.[73]

This standard would mean that LST of an incompetent—and by definition cognitively disabled—person could be forgone *if and only if* (1) the incompetent, prior to losing her mental capacity to make serious choices meaningfully, had refused the treatment in question under the factual circumstances she was now in, and (2) whoever was proposing to forgo treatment (typically a family member) would have to produce clear and convincing evidence of this refusal. Otherwise, treatment of the incompetent person would be legally and ethically mandatory, and there apparently would be no end to this obligation to provide LST other than presumably the proximate death of the incompetent or a showing that further treatment was itself unavoidably harmful to the incompetent.

If someone is incompetent to make an informed decision about accepting or refusing medical treatment, then someone else must decide what to do on his or her behalf. Traditionally, parents or guardians make these decisions for their minor children, and family members (sometimes close friends) make them for incompetent adults. It makes sense for someone personally close to and involved with the patient to make medical decisions on his or her behalf. Unlike strangers, such persons are much more likely to know and care about the patient and to genuinely have his or her own particular best interests at heart when making medical decisions. "Our common human experience informs us that family members . . . provide for the patient's comfort, care, and best interests . . . , and [it is] they who treat the patient as a person, rather than a symbol of a cause."[74] The Latin roots for "surrogate" reflect this as they can be translated as meaning "to ask near." When we cannot ask the person himself what treatment he wants or does not want, we ask someone as personally close to him as we can find.

The DRAs claim that the surrogates are not to be trusted as decision-makers for disabled persons. Diane Coleman has criticized surrogates as myopic in their valuation of the lives of the disabled and enmeshed in conflicts of interest:

> People with cognitive disabilities, like Terri Schiavo, cannot be fully and
> fairly represented by surrogates because of a conflict of interest inherent
> in the surrogacy relationship. Surrogates often value the lives of their
> wards far less than the wards value their own lives. Elder abuse is just
> one example of this. Some surrogates have a financial or other interest in
> hastening the ward's death.[75]

Although Coleman does not explain here what she means by the
assertion that close family members (spouses, parents, grandparents,
brothers, sisters) have an "inherent" conflict of interest when acting as
surrogates for their cognitively disabled relatives, a fair interpretation
of her position is that this conflict involves the surrogate's wish to get
rid of the responsibilities he or she has for the care of the disabled person by refusing LST for the disabled person and thereby eliminate her
and the burdens of caring for her at the same time. This interpretation
is buttressed by her statement that the responsible relatives value the
lives of their disabled relatives "far less" than the disabled value their
own lives. She also alludes to possible financial conflicts of interest—
that is, the surrogate's desire to inherit the disabled relative's property—
a charge that was frequently levied against Michael Schiavo. Coleman
and Gill have also argued that the reasons for distrusting family members and others as surrogates for the disabled goes much deeper:

> The courts have consistently excused parents who have murdered children
> with disabilities. . . . People with disabilities and incurable chronic
> diseases have experienced a long history of persecution and genocide. . . .
> [C]ontempt for life with disability is very much around us. . . . Physicians
> must not be given the power to decide who lives and who is escorted to
> death. As disabled historian Hugh Gallagher warns, the Nazi experience
> demonstrates how easily compassionate and well-educated physicians can
> lose their moral compass. . . . Medical rehabilitation specialists report that
> quadriplegics and other significantly disabled people are dying wrongfully
> in increasing numbers because emergency room physicians judge their
> quality of life as low and, therefore, withhold aggressive treatment. . . .
> Children with non-terminal disabilities who never asked to die are killed
> 'gently' by the denial of routine treatment. . . . The laws that protect our
> lives have often been the only buffer between us and annihilation.[76]

In this excerpt Coleman and Gill clearly imply that parents of disabled
children are not to be trusted because some undisclosed number of
them have murdered their children (i.e., killed them "gently" by denying them routine treatment). They also criticize physicians, who should
be a check on wrong decision making by surrogates, as "escort-
ing" the disabled to death like the Nazi doctors who participated in

the murder of disabled people even prior to the existence of the death camps.[77] They also suggest that "contempt for life with disability" thoroughly infects our society, including those family members who act as surrogates for their disabled loved ones and the physicians who treat disabled people.

Moreover, the DRAs believe that society's contempt for life with disability and the social devaluation of the life of persons with disabilities is so deep and pervasive that even the decision of a mentally competent disabled person to commit suicide (with or without someone else's help) or to refuse LST is morally coerced by the very limited options available to the disabled and should be considered invalid.[78] Notably, the DRAs have produced no "data showing that people with disabilities are more apt to end their lives than other classes of people."[79] The late Andrew Batavia, a co-author of the landmark Americans with Disability Act and a disability rights activist himself, observed "strong indications [exist] that a substantial majority of people with disabilities actually support a right to assisted dying," contrary to the claims of groups like Not Dead Yet.[80] Batavia also rejected on moral grounds the DRAs' claim that the disabled are too oppressed to choose for themselves:

> The general "oppressed minority" version of the personal assistance argument against assisted suicide is particularly offensive to people with disabilities who support the right. The contention that all people with disabilities are so oppressed, simply by virtue of their disability status, as to be presumed incapable of making end-of-life decisions reflects the same paternalism that the independent living movement was established to abolish.[81]

He sees the disability rights/independent living movement as based "fundamentally on autonomy" and urges that "people with disabilities should be allowed to make all decisions that affect their lives—including the decision to end their lives. . . ."[82] Anita Silvers, a philosopher who has written extensively on disability, rejects the DRA position as well:

> [D]espite acknowledging the systematic marginalization that people with disabilities endure, it seems wrong to think that having any kind of disability means being cognitively or psychologically disabled by society. To do so is to equate being disabled in any way with being globally debilitated.[83]

The literal and uniform application to all persons of the standard requiring clear and convincing evidence of the individual patient's wishes under the circumstances prior to forgoing LST is a truly radical proposal and would have two immediate and dramatic consequences.

First, all persons who were never competent—namely minor children and the developmentally disabled[84]—would have to receive LST; their parents, close relatives, or legally appointed surrogates would be prevented from deciding to forgo LST because these patients are and were unable to make any binding decisions about treatment at any point in their lives. They would become the "passive subjects of medical technology"[85] and would always have to receive LST, or perhaps at least be treated until their death is proximate regardless of the use of treatment because then and only then would the specter of contempt and bias in the treatment decisions have effectively passed.

Such a result would, of course, destroy a long tradition in both law and ethics of allowing involved and responsible parents to make medical decisions on behalf of their minor children if these decisions are not clearly contrary to the best interests of the child in question. Although parental medical decision-making authority is not unlimited (they are not permitted to refuse clearly beneficial treatment for their child for any reason, religious or otherwise), the law and ethics have considered them to have the inherent right and responsibility to make medical decisions for their children as the ones best suited by love, knowledge, and attachment to direct the course of their children's lives. No evidence exists that parents routinely or commonly abuse their children, whether disabled or not, by denying them beneficial medical treatment. To be sure, some parents do make bad or ill-motivated decisions about medical treatment for their children that should not be honored, but these are already prohibited by law, and health care professionals are legally bound to report them to state authorities.[86] The DRAs have not made a convincing case why this tradition, and the set of values it assumes, should be set aside for minor children.

Many persons who become developmentally disabled while minors survive until majority age. Once they reach majority age, the medical decision-making authority of their parents legally ends. Consequently, the clear and convincing evidence standard as proposed by the DRAs would have to be applied to them as it would to all other adults. Therefore, in the absence of the proper evidence of individuals' wishes about treatment (which would necessarily be the case as they would almost surely lack the mental capacity to make their own decisions), they would have to be treated in all cases. Elsewhere I have argued at some length that developmentally disabled persons have several important interests at stake when receiving medical treatment: (1) in being free of pain and suffering unrelated to a compensating benefit; (2) in being treated as unique individuals (not as some generic and anonymous "disabled person") who have a personal history, individual character, and particular wants and needs; (3) in not being subjected to invasive medical treatment that is unduly burdensome or nonbeneficial; and (4) in having a meaningful quality of life relative to them as individuals.[87] In order to respect individuals who are developmentally disabled like all other individual persons, these interests need to be protected and preserved through the right to give or withhold informed consent to treatment as exercised by a concerned and involved surrogate:

> Those bearing the responsibility to act as surrogates for those who cannot speak for themselves surely must recognize that the developmentally disabled historically have been the subjects of misunderstandings, inattention, prejudgment, and outright bias in the delivery of health care (and other human services). But this history should not strip responsible surrogates of their ability to exercise a developmentally disabled person's right to give or withhold consent to treatment. Instead, it underscores the importance of such decisions being exercised carefully and deliberately.[88]

The DRAs' position would deprive developmentally disabled persons of their right to have a careful, appropriate, and individualized decision made on their behalf, one that would be aimed at protecting their personal interests, not the interests of the surrogate, society, or anyone else.

Second, the application of the clear and convincing evidence standard to adults who were formerly competent will surely result in treatment being imposed in the overwhelming majority of cases because very few people will have expressed themselves clearly and precisely enough to satisfy the extremely demanding nature of the standard. For someone like Terri Schiavo to satisfy it, she would have had to have left nearly indisputable, reliable evidence that she would refuse gastrostomy tube feeding when she was diagnosed as being permanently unconscious (and this puts aside the question of whether she would have to predict the extreme controversy within her family over her condition and prior expression of wishes). This requires foresight no one has, and no one can reasonably be expected to have it. The strict application of the clear and convincing standard imposes on persons the risks of treatment, of invasions of the body, and of depersonalization, dangers that are just as grave as the risk of denying treatment. This standard has been heavily criticized for these and other reasons in the bioethics literature and by the courts.[89]

In my view, the DRAs' insistence on the application of the clear and convincing evidence standard again directly flows from their core convictions. They see this standard, despite its radical nature and far-reaching implications for millions, as necessary to protect the disabled from the apparently vicious, murderous prejudice of mainstream society, medicine, bioethics, and even the very families of the disabled themselves. While no one should dispute the history of shameful treatment of the disabled in this country, it is unjustified for the DRAs to claim that even the families of disabled people are so steeped in prejudice that they cannot be trusted at all to be loyal to the best interests of their disabled relatives. The clearly better solution is for everyone involved in decisions to forgo LST to watch carefully for bad decisions and object to them rather than to routinely force treatment on everyone in nearly every case.

It is likewise simply implausible to assert that society in general and the medical profession and bioethicists in particular are engaged in systematic efforts to eliminate the disabled that can be overcome only by enforcing a standard that eliminates surrogate decision making and forces treatment onto nearly everyone. The formerly competent will almost always be treated because so relatively few persons complete advance directives that are available for use when the time comes, or leave clear and convincing evidence of their wishes that will specify the precise factual circumstances they will be in. Children and the developmentally disabled will have to be treated in all cases. In short, the DRAs' position virtually eliminates the right to refuse treatment for the incompetent. "This is a regime of rights turned on its head. It is a demand for so much formality and specificity, ultimately for the fulfillment of such impossible conditions, that the right [to refuse] vanishes. It vanishes because real life has no place in [this] vision."[90] Every individual, whether disabled or not, deserves an individualized decision about LST to be made on the particular merits and circumstances of his or her own case. It is truly anomalous, even perverse, for the DRAs to insist upon a uniform result for all disabled people—even the disabled who are mentally competent and can express their own wishes just like the nondisabled—while harshly criticizing those who do not treat disabled people as discrete, valuable individuals.

:: Conclusion

A different interpretation of the DRAs' position in the Schiavo case might see it as shrewdly practical and political: It is the only way they can (1) really demonstrate the point that one cannot fairly evaluate or understand disability from the position of the "perfectly" able-bodied (recall Koch's provocative notion that we are *all* "incomplete and unable"), and (2) hope to create sufficient public support for an alternative way of social management of disability—one committed to allocating resources to reasonably maximize every individual's capacity to experience and interact with his or her world. Perhaps the DRAs have so few venues in which they can effectively and widely broadcast their very real and substantial distress over the situation of the disabled in America that they could not pass up the opportunity to latch themselves onto Terri Schiavo's national prominence and use it to advance their project to change the oppression of the disabled.[91] Perhaps able-bodied people consistently and drastically underestimate the depth of antagonism and bias they harbor against the disabled more than they could possibly grasp.

While we all should be sympathetic to these goals and work to root out the "better dead than disabled" attitude that does exist in our midst, we should *not* accept the way the DRAs (and others, such as certain politicians) hijacked the Terri Schiavo tragedy and used it for their own purposes—none of which had anything to do with her personally. Ms. Schiavo was not treated unjustly because she was disabled. Her husband, the Florida judges involved in her case, and the Federal judges who refused to overturn the results of the extensive litigation in the state courts (at the ill-advised invitation of the U.S. Congress) did not treat her as the object of prejudice, contempt, and disrespect due to her disability. This was the wrong case for the DRAs to use to highlight their agenda of social and political change of the way disability is thought about and disabled people are treated. Highly questionable conceptions of disability, distortion of facts, and advocacy of unrealistic and unfair standards for surrogate decision making about life-sustaining medical treatment should not be employed to advance even the important and necessary goals of improving the lives of the members of our family, church, synagogue, mosque, neighborhood, or community who happen to be disabled.

NOTES TO CHAPTER 8

1. 1. Various organizations. Issues surrounding Terri Schindler-Schiavo are disability rights issues, say national disability organizations. Available at http://www.raggededgemagazine.com/schiavostatement.html. The organizations listed as signers of this statement are ADA Watch, ADAPT, AIMMM—Advancing Independence, Center for Self-Determination,

Center for Human Policy, Citizens United Resisting Euthanasia (CURE), Disability Rights Center, Disability Rights Education & Defense Fund, Disability Rights Project of the Public Interest Law Center of Philadelphia, Hospice Patients Alliance, National Catholic Partnership on Disability, National Coalition for Disability Rights, National Coalition on Self-Determination, National Council on Independent Living, National Disabled Students Union, National Down Syndrome Congress, National Organization on Disability, National Spinal Cord Injury Association, Not Dead Yet, Self Advocates Becoming Empowered (SABE), TASH, World Association of Persons with disAbilities, and World Institute on Disability.

2. Ibid.

3. See Dworkin, R. The rights of Alan Bakke. In J. Arthur, ed., *Morality and Moral Controversies*, 6th ed., Saddle River, N.J.: Prentice Hall, 2002, p. 521.

4. Koch, T. The ideology of normalcy. *Journal of Disability Policy Studies* 2005;16(2):123–129. While I am not at all persuaded that the values inherent in the ideology of normalcy are in fact endorsed by most bioethicists and used by them as Koch claims, his distinction will nevertheless by useful in trying to understand the meaning of disability in the Schiavo case.

5. Koch also sees them expressing their values "through different vocabularies and powered by different logics," Normalcy, p. 123. As I am primarily interested in the differences in values here, I will not explicitly delve much into the differences in vocabulary or logic.

6. All quotations in this paragraph are from Koch, "Normalcy," p. 124.

7. All quotations in this paragraph are from "Normalcy," pp. 123, 124, and 126. I have not included Koch's references to Darwin and competition in his exposition of the ideology of normalcy as I find them morally irrelevant and distracting.

8. Amundson, R., and Taira, G. Our lives and ideologies. The effect of life experience on the perceived morality of the policy of physician-assisted suicide. *Journal of Disability Policy Studies* 2005;16:54.

9. Saxton, M. Why members of the disability community oppose prenatal diagnosis and selective abortion. In E. Parens and A. Asch, eds. *Prenatal Testing and Disability Rights*, Washington D.C.: Georgetown University Press, 2000, p. 149.

10. DRA statement (emphasis added).

11. Bickenbach, J.E. Disability and life-ending decisions. In M. Battin, R. Rhodes, and A. Silvers, eds. *Physician Assisted Suicide: Expanding the Debate*, New York: Routledge, 1998, pp. 131–132.

12. Coleman, D., and Gill, C. Testimony before the Constitution Subcommittee of the Judiciary Committee of the U.S. House of Representatives, April 29, 1996. Available at http://www.notdeadyet.org/docs/house1.html.

13. Cited in Steinbock, B. Disability, prenatal testing, and selective abortion. In Parens and Asch, *Prenatal Testing*, p. 113 (emphasis deleted).

14. Ibid., p. 114.

15. "Report of Autopsy" by Jon R. Thogmartin, Chief Medical Examiner, District Six, Pasco & Pinellas Counties, June 13, 2005; supporting report of Stephen Nelson, M.D., designated consultant neuropathologist, p. 5. Available under the Timeline entry for June 15, 2005, at http://www.miami.edu/ethics/schiavo/schiavo_timeline.html.

16. Ibid., Nelson report.

17. Ibid., p. 2.

18. "Report of Autopsy," p. 1.

19. Multi-Society Task Force on PVS. Medical aspects of the persistent vegetative state (first of two parts). *New England Journal of Medicine* 1994;330:1499–1508; Multi-Society Task Force on PVS. Medical aspects of the persistent vegetative state (second of two parts). *New England Journal of Medicine* 1994;330:1572–1579.

20. Cranford, R. Facts, lies, and videotapes: the permanent vegetative state and the sad case of Terri Schiavo. *Journal of Law, Medicine & Ethics* 2005;33(2):365.

21. *The American Heritage Dictionary of the English Language*, 4th ed., 2000. Available at http://dictionary.reference.com/search?q=disability.

22. "Florida Bioethics Leaders' Analysis of HB 701," March 7 & 10, 2005 (emphasis in original). Available under the March 7, 2005, Timeline entry at http://www.miami.edu/ethics/schiavo/schiavo_timeline.html.

23. Rachels, J. *The End of Life*. Oxford: Oxford University Press, 1986, p. 5.

24. Amundson and Taira, "Life Experience," p. 54.

25. DRAs Statement. I believe they are intentionally adding "Schindler" to her name as a rhetorical device to associate her more closely with her parents, who were adopting the same positions as the DRAs, including the manifestly false views that Ms. Schiavo was not permanently unconscious and that she had not received proper rehabilitation. These are discussed below in much greater detail.

26. Quoted in Eisenberg, J.B. *Using Terri: The Religious Right's Conspiracy to Take Away Our Rights*. New York: HarperCollins, 2005, p. 70.

27. All quotations in this paragraph are from DRAs' Statement (emphasis added).

28. Wertz, D., and Fletcher, J.C. A critique of some feminist challenges to prenatal diagnosis. *Journal of Women's Health* 1993;2(2):175.

29. Ackerman, F. Assisted suicide, terminal illness, severe disability, and the double standard. In Batttin, Rhodes, and Silvers. *Expanding the Debate*, p. 154, citing disability rights activist Cyndi Jones.

30. Steinbock, "Prenatal Testing," p. 112.

31. Ibid., pp. 112–113.

32. Under California criminal law, for example, such conduct would undoubtedly violate Penal Code §245 (2005) which prohibits any assault with deadly weapon or by force likely to produce great bodily injury and punishes such behavior by "by imprisonment in the state prison for two, three, or four years, or in a county jail for not exceeding one year, or by a fine not exceeding ten thousand dollars ($10,000), or by both the fine and imprisonment." The victim could also sue for civil damages as well.

33. Asch, A. Reproductive technology and disability. In S. Cohen and N. Taub, eds. *Reproductive Laws for the 1990s*. Clifton, N.J.: Humana Press, 1989, p. 73.

34. I am very reluctant to distinguish "normal" people from "disabled" people, as doing so seems to endorse the preposterous notion that disabled people cannot be normal. I oppose any use of language that even suggests persons with disabilities are of any lesser moral status or possess any less moral worth or dignity than persons lacking a disability or impairment.

35. Silvers, A. Protecting the innocents from physician-assisted suicide. In Battin, Rhodes, and Silvers, *Expanding the Debate*, p. 139.

36. Kuczewski, M.G. Disability: An agenda for bioethics. *American Journal of Bioethics* 2001;1(3):139.

37. Amundson and Taira, "Life Experience," p. 54.

38. E.g., Batavia, A.I. Disability and physician-assisted dying. In T.E. Quill and M.P. Battin, eds. *Physician-Assisted Dying: The Case for Palliative Care & Patient Choice*. Baltimore: Johns Hopkins University Press, 2004, p. 57; and Kuczewski, "Agenda for Bioethics," p. 41.

39. For example, Alice Mailhot, without any qualification or limitation, calls bioethicists "the most dangerous people in the U.S. today . . . 'way above skinheads, whose beliefs they appear to share." Her article is titled "Bioethics: theories from hell" and is available on the Not Dead Yet Website at http://www.notdeadyet.org/docs/bioethic.html.

40. DRAs' Statement.

41. Brief of *Amicus Curiae* Not Dead Yet et al. In Support of Appellants and Requesting Reversal, February 21, 2003. Available at http://www.notdeadyet.org/docs/schaivobrief.html.

42. DRAs' Statement.

43. Coleman in Eisenberg, p. 73.

44. Brief *Amicus Curiae* of International Task Force on Euthanasia & Assisted Suicide in Support of Appellant/Petitioners, (undated), pp. 9, 19. Available at http://www.internationaltaskforce.org/pdf/schiavo.pdf.

45. *In re Schiavo*, Circuit Court for Pinellas County, Florida, Probate Division, No. 90–2908GD-003, Order, February 11, 2000, p. 6 (emphasis added).

46. Under the usual legal rules, an appellate court is obligated to affirm the trial court's determinations of disputed facts, such as Ms. Schiavo's medical condition, whenever substantial evidence supports those determinations.

47. *In re Schiavo*, 780 So.2d 176, 177 (Fla. Ct. App. 2001 (Schiavo I) (emphasis added).

48. *In re Schiavo*, 792 So.2d 551, 560 (Fla. Ct. App. 2001 (Schiavo II) (emphasis added).

49. *In re Schiavo*, 800 So.2d 640, 643–644 (Fla. Ct. App. 2001 (Schiavo III).

50. Ibid., p. 644, 646 (emphasis added).

51. Ibid.

52. Ibid., p. 646.

53. The Court of Appeal noticed his absence too: "However, Dr. Webber, who was so critical in this court's decision to remand the case, made no further appearance in these proceedings." *In re Schiavo*, 851 So.2d 182, 184 (Fla. Ct. App. 2003 (Schiavo IV).

54. *In re Schiavo*, Circuit Court for Pinellas County, Florida, Probate Division, No. 90–2908GD-003, Order, November 22, 2002 (emphasis added).

55. Ibid.

56. "Perhaps the most compelling testimony was that of Dr. Bambakidis who explained to the court the agony and soul-searching which he underwent to arrive at his opinion that Terry Schiavo is in a persistent vegetative state. He concluded that *all the data as a whole supports permanent vegetative state.*" Ibid. (emphasis added).

57. Cranford, "Facts, lies," pp. 366–369; cf. "A Common Uniqueness: Medical Facts in the Schiavo Case" (in this volume).

58. *Schiavo IV*, p. 185.

59. Ibid., p. 186.

60. DRAs' Statement.

61. HB 35-E, Florida Statutes Chapter 41. This statute was struck down as unconstitutional in *Bush v. Schiavo*, 885 So.2d 321 (Fla. 2004) because it violated the separation of powers and made an improper delegation of legislative authority to the governor.

62. Wolfson, J. A Report to Governor Jeb Bush, In the Matter of Theresa Marie Schiavo, December 1, 2003. Available under the Timeline entry for December 1, 2003, at http://www.miami.edu/ethics/schiavo/schiavo_timeline.html.

63. Ibid., p. 2.

64. Ibid., p. 8.

65. Ibid., pp. 8, 9. The autopsy report (p. 32) confirms that "intense rehabilitation" occurred while she was at the Mediplex facility.

66. Wolfson report, p. 9.

67. DRAs' Statement.

68. Autopsy report, *passim*.

69. See *In Re: Rosebush*, No. 88–349180-AZ (Oakland County Cir. Ct., July 29, 1988), *In Re: Jobes*, 529 A.2d 434, 438–440 (N.J. 1987).

70. DRAs' Statement.

71. Not Dead Yet *amicus* brief.

72. Ibid.

73. *Conservatorship of Wendland*, 26 Cal 4th 519 (2001); Brief *Amicus Curiae* of the National Legal Center for the Medically Dependent & Disabled, Inc. in Support of Respondents Florence Wendland and Rebekah Vinson, filed in the California Supreme Court, October 27, 2000, p. 13.

74. *In re Jobes*, 529 A.2d 434, 445 (N.J. 1987).

75. Coleman in Eisenberg, p. 69.

76. Coleman, D., and Gill, C. The disability rights opposition to physician-assisted suicide. In J. McDonald, ed. *Contemporary Moral Issues in a Diverse Society*. Belmont, Calif.: Wadsworth, 1998, pp. 197, 198, 199, 200.

77. Lifton, R. *The Nazi Doctors*. New York: Basic Books, 1986, pp. 45–79.

78. Bickenbach, "Disability," pp. 123–132.
79. Silvers in Battin, Rhodes, and Silvers, *Expanding the Debate*, pp. 139–140.
80. Batavia, "Physician-Assisted Dying," pp. 57, 61–62. Mr. Batavia died in 2003 at the age of 45. He was a quadriplegic who used a wheelchair after an auto accident at the age of 16.
81. Ibid., p. 67.
82. Ibid., p. 63.
83. Silvers in Battin, Rhodes, and Silvers, *Expanding the Debate*, p. 142.
84. "Developmental disability" usually refers to a disability that originates before an individual reaches 18 years old, can be expected to continue indefinitely, and constitutes a substantial disability for that individual. It includes conditions such as mental retardation, cerebral palsy, epilepsy, and autism.
85. *Conservatorship of Drabick*, 245 Cal. Rptr. 840, 854 (Ct. App. 1988).
86. All states have laws forbidding child abuse and neglect, including medical neglect, and all states require medical professionals to report child abuse and neglect to appropriate authorities.
87. Nelson, L.J. Respect for the developmentally disabled and forgoing life-sustaining treatment. *Mental Retardation and Developmental Disabilities Research Reviews* 2003;9:3–9.
88. Ibid., pp. 3–4.
89. See, for example, Wolf, S.M. Nancy Beth Cruzan: In no voice at all. *Hastings Center Report* 1990;20(1):38–41; and Eisenberg, "Using Terri."
90. Wolf, "Cruzan," p. 39.
91. I owe these ideas to Michelle Oberman of the Santa Clara University Law School.

9 ::

Framing Terri Schiavo: Gender, Disability, and Fetal Protection

Robin N. Fiore

For more than a decade, Theresa Marie Schiavo's family members fought to control her care, involving not only state and federal courts, but also Florida's Legislature and chief executive, and, ultimately, the Congress and the President of United States.[1] While the blogosphere hyperventilated, ethicists, health care providers, and legal professionals issued calls for universal advance care planning. Meanwhile, the Roman Catholic Church and legislators in a number of states sought to limit the kinds of medical interventions to which such advance directives could apply. The central issue—the right to refuse unwanted medical intervention, including life-sustaining treatment—was "resolved" by the courts; although the right to refuse remains intact, we are no closer to a social consensus about "permitting death to take place unopposed."[2]

At bottom, Schiavo[3] is, indeed, an extreme instance of family disagreement about medical care. It has been described as the most litigated case in United States legal history, and it is therefore not surprising that analyses have concentrated on the abundant legal and political issues, overlooking what I take to be a second Schiavo front in the public arena: namely, an argument concerning women's equality and moral agency. The debate consisted of the deployment of a series of competing frames in which the organization of the facts of the case tacitly promoted conclusions about matters that either were not articulated or were disguised in the legal contest—in particular, questions of gender. Although gender was not explicitly addressed in the legal proceedings,[4] the public framing of Schiavo was heavily infused with imagery, stereotypes, and associations through which gender surreptitiously entered the debate.

In this chapter, I consider Schiavo from the perspective of its gender implications. "Gender," as I use it here, refers to contingent and historical relations of power between the sexes.[5] Men and women are both gendered, but are gendered differently. That is, men-as-a-group and women-as-a-group are differently situated with respect to social power and privilege, status and respect, and access to social resources (e.g., health care). Nothing essential is implied about "the way men [women] are" and there is no claim that the power differentials are attributable to all members, or to only members, of a group constituted by gender. Nevertheless, socially constructed attributes persisting over long periods may become so deeply associated with the groups so constituted that one may analyze the implications of that attribute for the group in question, while rejecting its inevitability.[6] With that understanding, an analysis of gender need not be regarded as either incoherent or stigmatizing.

In what follows, I offer an analysis of the public debate through the consideration of three salient frames: the gender frame, the disability rights frame, and the fetal protection frame. Although each portrays a very different understanding of what was at stake in Schiavo, each frame implicitly and significantly calls into question the moral agency of women. Consequently, in my view, no matter which frame was ascendant at the conclusion of the Schiavo case, women-as-a-group lost ground. Despite the fact that a nominal "right to let die"[7] was affirmed, the long, rancorous public debate on end-of-life care has the potential to diminish women's ability to effectively exercise autonomy in the future.

∷ Framing: Proposing a Perspective

Frame analysis describes a wide range of approaches that endeavor to explain the role of communication in how humans organize experience. Most simply, frames can be understood as "thought organizers"—basic cognitive structures that determine which parts of reality are noticed. As Todd Gitlin puts it, "Frames are principles of selection, emphasis, presentation composed of little tacit theories about what exists, what happens, and what matters."[8]

Framing theory originated in the insight that a message is a complex, comprising information bound together with a suggested pattern for its integration.[9] Moreover, our receipt of a message has the potential to reorganize our experience and remake our receptivity to future messages. Accordingly, the adoption of any particular frame depends, to some extent, on an appeal that is internal to the message and is inseparable from it. On this view, words or concepts that are tightly bound to deep-seated cultural associations carry meanings that are not strictly a function of literality, meanings that resist being consciously recognized, attended to, and reflected upon: for example, to the extent that pernicious racial, ethnic, and other epithets are inseparable from historical context, they may prove recalcitrant to reclamation.[10]

In applied contexts, such as political science and communications, theories of framing are deployed in analyses of persuasion. In those fields, frame receptivity is understood as a matter of choice: framing is an active process of selecting words, images, and context to manipulate or manage the ways in which people think about issues.[11] Framing is not merely "spin" or choosing more appealing words (e.g., "personal accounts" in lieu of "private accounts" in the Social Security debates[12]); framing shifts contexts in order to change the moral valence. The goal is to reorient, to establish a different value ordering or moral scheme, to reset the problematic. For example, changing the frame from "domestic spying program" to "terrorist surveillance program" changes the set of relevant moral concerns and their ordering. While referring to the same policy, the two frames offer competing conceptualizations of the moral issues. Similarly, changing frames from "estate tax" to "death tax" reconfigures the set of stakeholders and the receiver's personal connection to the policy.

The goal of framing, then, is to influence how a particular moral problem is understood and even to induce a certain conclusion. Competing frames propose different perspectives from which to evaluate an issue, each of which is intended to preclude certain conclusions and promote others by privileging certain elements. Thus, the adoption of a frame forces "a particular problem definition, causal interpretation, moral evaluation, and/or treatment recommendation."[13]

Controversial ethico-political problems with compound or complex considerations and incommensurable potential solutions, such as those in bioethics, provide rich opportunities for framing contests. Framing theory suggests that it is not the solutions that are weighed and judged as much as it is the frames themselves. Furthermore, an individual's response to a particular frame is conditioned; it is contingent upon previously endorsed values and commitments. In competitions, the successful frame is one that invokes a value toward which a person is already generally predisposed. The most successful frames attach to identity conferring commitments, the broad themes and ideals by which individuals organize and make sense of their moral choices and experiences. For example, if a policy or solution is posed within a justice frame, it is appealing to the extent that the responder has already adopted a view in which justice claims are compelling. Framing may also invoke preexisting attitudes regarding either the disputing parties or the institutions or organizations strongly affiliated with one of the frames. For example, in Schiavo, attitudes toward the medical profession and bioethicists ("biodeathicists") are implicated in the disability rights frame.

Receiver ambivalence plays an important role in determining whether a frame succeeds in recruiting adherents.[14] It is not uncommon for individuals to experience conflicts in thinking about complex moral problems, especially problems where the competition is between moral values or moral systems that are comparably compelling or worthy. For example, on the question of abortion, it would not be unusual to find within a single person both of the following considerations: (a) personal values opposed to the taking of life and (b) empathy and/or political solidarity with those who are affected by the issue and have different needs/lives/views. Similarly, on the issue of physician-aid-in-dying, a person might hold (a) that it is wrong for physicians to hasten dying, and (b) that people should be able to choose how and when they die. In contrast, less ambivalent individuals or "true believers" filter out frames that are incompatible with their beliefs and commitments and are thus less susceptible to recruitment.

Returning now to Schiavo, the three frames discussed below may shed light on why clinical and Constitutional considerations offered in other venues had so little impact on the public and on the politics surrounding this case.

∷ Gender Frame: Sleeping Beauty and Lifetime TV

The Schiavo narrative shares many features with landmark "right-to-die" cases involving catastrophic brain injury, not the least of which is that the tragic central figure is an attractive, young, white woman. Just as media attention to missing persons skews to those who are attractive, young, white, and female, so too have commentators identified a similar "Missing White Woman Syndrome" in medical cases. As the physician-bioethicist Steven Miles points out, "the plights of injured young women are more likely to engage the public and attract right-to-life advocates."[15] The pensive yearbook photo of an attractive young Karen Ann Quinlan led the media and the public to picture her "as a sort of tragic Sleeping Beauty."[16] Thus represented, she waits for rescue. The gendered imagery is not merely whimsical. The familiar mode of rescue—a "miraculous awakening"—may help to explain the apparent over-representation of females in cases opposing the withdrawal of life support.

The Sleeping Beauty metaphor is also suggestive with respect to women's "overtreatment" at the end of life relative to men.[17] Feminist analyses of right-to-die cases concur that deeply embedded cultural associations of the female with passivity and the male with agency and activity may lead to gendered distinctions in quality-of-life assessments. Diane Raymond concludes that the embrace of a higher standard of quality of life for men may contribute to "keeping dying, suffering women alive."[18] Dena Davis argues that the cultural valorization of women's self-sacrifice gives rise to social expectations that, for the sake of others, women should forego acting on interests they may have in relieving their suffering by hastening death.[19] These expectations pressure women to protect relatives who might appear uncaring if they did not insist on "everything" being done, uphold respect for life, and enable others to obtain meaning or benefit from their continued existence. In contrast, Susan M. Wolf and others worry that normative ideals of feminine self-sacrifice and passivity might lead to physicians or policy makers' eagerness—rather than reluctance—to permit (voluntary) physician-assisted suicide.[20] The apparent disagreement about what follows from sexist stereotypes underscores the fact that gender is inflected by other privileging or disadvantaging social identities as well as by economic and familial resources. Rather than disempowering all women for the sake of protecting the less privileged or least well off, the focus should be on fashioning just social arrangements.

Gendered norms of femininity as well as women's experience of early and lifelong responsibilities for caregiving are often presumed to render the physical dependency and immobility associated with illness more tolerable for women. Thus, the acceptable benefit/burden ratio of life-sustaining medical technology and intuitions about its (in)appropriateness follow a similarly gender-inflected pattern. According to a study of the judicial reasoning in right-to-die cases by Steven Miles and Alison August,[21] life-support-dependent males are perceived as "subjected to assault;" for females, however, such measures are forms of aid to the vulnerable that, if withheld, would constitute "medical neglect." Despite gender-neutral policies affirming the right to refuse life-sustaining treatment, the Miles and August study reveals gender-patterned attitudes that result in substantively unequal treatment of similarly situated adult males and females. For example, in cases involving previously competent patients without advance directives, the study found that courts were willing to construct the "patient's preference" from the memories and insights of family and friends in the case of males (6 out of 8)—even when that constructed preference supported the termination of life-sustaining treatment—but significantly less willing in the case of females (only 2 out of 14).[22]

Miles and August enumerate the ways in which judges in end-of-life cases invoked gender stereotypes and rendered different decisions depending on the patient's sex. First, many courts characterized statements made by male patients regarding end-of-life preferences as "rational" and regarded them as "matters of conviction." In contrast, the female patients' preferences were characterized as "unreflective," "emotional," or "immature;" their statements were discounted as mere "reactions" or expressions of "distaste." Second, courts failed to acknowledge women's moral agency by ignoring patterns of conduct (avoidance of the medical care system, consistency of statements over time) that were taken as characteristic and dispositive for males, in effect treating females without explicit advance directives—but not similarly situated males—as if they had never been competent. Moreover, as the study notes, courts explicitly claimed a parental role only in relation to females (Quinlan, Cruzan); such a role was specifically rejected in the case of a male (Brophy). Finally, courts applied different standards of evidence: in constructing men's preferences, the courts accepted remote discussions and evidence derived from third-party assessments of character as sufficient for "substituted judgment" but rejected similarly nonspecific or casual remarks by women, citing the need to "shelter" them from greedy family members or adverting to the risks of relying on women's casual statements when life was at stake.[23]

The Miles and August study predates the Schiavo litigation. Both Nancy Cruzan and Terri Schiavo were reported to have expressed their wishes to family members in similarly casual language. Florida found such statements sufficiently clear and convincing; 15 years earlier, in the case of Cruzan, Missouri did not. It would be interesting to know whether that difference can be attributed to differences in state constitutions, or changes in attitudes toward women's agency (locally or more broadly), or merely the particularities of the two cases. Although the Florida court's decision to allow the termination of life-sustaining treatment was based on acceptance of the "constructed preference" proposed by Michael Schiavo (Terri Schiavo's husband), it is discouraging to note that those on both sides invoked many of the gender-patterned attitudes noted above and expressed themselves in ways that compromised Terri Schiavo's dignity. A representative blogger wrote: "Can you imagine tearful parents [of a married, 40-year-old man] appealing to the United States Congress to 'Please save our little boy?'"[24] At the other end of the literary spectrum, Joan Didion—award-winning novelist, essayist, journalist, and playwright—disparaged then-competent Terri Schiavo regarding the style of the oral statements she is alleged to have uttered ("hearsay") after watching a television movie about a young, female PVS patient with a feeding tube (Quinlan). Didion wrote:

> Imagine it. You are in your early twenties. You are watching a movie, say, on Lifetime, in which someone has a feeding tube. You pick up an empty chip bowl. "No tubes for me," you say as you get up to fill it. What are the chances you have given this even a passing thought?[25]

Elements of class as well as gender disrespect are apparent in Didion's reconstruction of the scene, with its references to "potato chips" and to "Lifetime TV"—which markets itself specifically as "television for women."[26]

Regardless of whether one agrees with the Schiavo court's acceptance of the reports of Terri Schiavo's wishes or the ultimate outcome of the case, it is not at all implausible to attribute the public acrimony in part to the persistence of gender valuations that discount women's capacity for moral reasoning. One mode of devaluation is the privileging of detached moral judgments and abstract styles of moral expression, as reflected in Susan M. Wolf's criticism of "the [Cruzan] court's fantasy of a world in which people speak contract-talk about their death. . . ."[27] Related concerns reverberate in the suggestion that the insistence on lawyerly language to express one's last wishes discourages more widespread utilization of advance directives.

Schiavo has been credited with generating unprecedented interest in health care advance directives as a means to preserve personal preferences regarding end-of-life care from misinterpretation or annulment by family members, professionals, or civil officials. Gender-based power imbalances (as well as other relations of power not addressed here) simultaneously affect individuals' willingness to participate in advance care planning and the likelihood that advance directives will be honored. While the empirical data are not conclusive, there is wide-ranging support for the view that women are differently situated than men with respect to health care and the legal system and that they may experience diminished agency in health care decision making *in virtue of gender.*[28]

The most obvious gender-specific issue relates to pregnancy. A pregnant woman has fewer rights to terminate life support or refuse care than a man or a woman who is not pregnant. Only four states explicitly permit a woman to refuse life support if she is pregnant. In states with living will statutes, 32 of 47 limit the applicability of living wills if a woman is pregnant, explicitly prohibiting the termination of life support whether or not the fetus is viable.[29] Such provisions are tantamount to declaring pregnant women incompetent. Sixteen states explicitly forbid health care surrogates from ordering the withholding of life support on behalf of pregnant patients; five permit a woman to specify whether her surrogate can do so in the event that she is pregnant. Even in jurisdictions where there is no specific pregnancy suspension, historical precedents make it more reasonable to anticipate that courts will treat a pregnant woman differently than a man or a woman who is not pregnant.[30]

In policies in which there is no specific reference to women or pregnancy, women's right to refuse medical interventions can be at risk through the operation of more general gender disadvantage. The first draft of the Maryland Health Care Decisions Act of 1993 included a provision that would require the sole provider of a minor child to obtain court approval before refusing life support. The impact of such a provision would fall mostly on women because the majority of sole providers of minor children are women; the gender-neutral language serves to render the differential impact invisible. In fact, the burden of the draft provision would have fallen most heavily on Maryland's significant population of women suffering from end-stage HIV/AIDS if public comments had not resulted in the elimination of this provision from the final version.[31]

The point here is that reliance on living wills is inadequate. Living wills cannot address implicit gender disparities in the health care system or the attitudes that contribute to dignitary harms as well as to poorer clinical outcomes for women.[32] It is often suggested that the durable power of attorney is a more reliable way to ensure that an individual's advance directives are honored. Although I am sympathetic to such a view, reliance on durable power of attorney may prove inadequate if some disability rights advocates succeed in their attempts to undermine surrogate decision via substituted judgment.

A more urgent threat to the right to refuse unwanted medical interventions is posed by state legislative activity on end-of-life decision-making issues generated by the Schiavo case. Many states are considering measures to limit the right to refuse certain kinds of medical interventions and to limit physicians' reliance on patients' oral statements. In connection with its Schiavo advocacy, National Right to Life (NRLC) is promoting a "Model Starvation and Dehydration of Persons with Disabilities Prevention Act" that will result in the continuance of medically supplied nutrition and hydration in incapacitated persons in most instances.[33] In order to refuse medically supplied nutrition and hydration, the Model Act requires patients to execute written advance directives with a kind of specificity that would be possible only if a patient and physician had foreseen and discussed the future state of medical technology and the patient's precise future condition and treatment. Moreover, the Model Act reduces the powers of court-appointed guardians, eliminates the "best interest" standard of proxy decision making regarding medically supplied nutrition and hydration, and thwarts the goals of hospice care.

All of those implications are particularly relevant for women, given their greater reliance on living wills.[34] Women constitute the largest percentage of the very old and those with irreversible acute cognitive impairment. Unlike PVS patients such as Terri Schiavo, those elderly patients *can* suffer pain, discomfort, fear, and confusion. Critics of the "best interests" *qua* objective standard for surrogate decision making have identified ways in which the standard needs improvement, but the "best interests" standard remains an essential protection for the vulnerable against needless suffering inflicted for the sake of politics or financial gain.[35]

:: The Disability Rights Frame

The "first wave" of the disability rights movement focused primarily on issues related to integrating people with disabilities into the mainstream of society, such as modifications to infrastructure, access to technology, and the social provision of personal care needs. On the central moral issues of abortion, reproductive technology, and euthanasia, disability advocates take a variety of positions and work though dozens of separate organizations. Some worry about unjustified paternalism and infringements of choice in dying; others worry that if certain kinds of choices become socially acceptable—abortion of impaired fetuses, assistance in dying—they will become social imperatives rather than choices. Tension exists between aspirations for self-determination and concerns about the cumulative social impact of individual choices. Despite differences, disability advocates strongly object to decisions' being based on non-disabled people's assumptions that life with a disability is not worth living. Disability advocates are, therefore, typically critical of substituted judgment, holding that human adaptability and the likelihood of technological progress preclude reliance on the past statements of formerly competent, formerly able patients.

In the United States, in the 30 years since the Quinlan decision, tension between the ethical principles of patient autonomy and beneficence has resolved in favor of patient self-determination. Likewise, the primacy of patients' own understandings of their good has become the broadly endorsed ground for the discussion and resolution of end-of-life decisions. The Florida Constitution contains an explicit right of privacy: "Every natural person has the right to be let alone and free from governmental intrusion into the person's private life except as otherwise provided herein."[36] In 1990, the Florida Supreme Court[37] effectively recognized a (state) constitutional right of patients to refuse medical interventions, including those without which life would cease, when the patient has expressed those desires either in a living will, through oral declarations, or by the written designation of a health care proxy. Furthermore, the state may not override the clearly expressed wishes of a patient to be disconnected from a feeding tube. Thus, since 1990, the same year Terri Schiavo sustained her injury, Floridians have had the strongest legal assurance that unwanted medical interventions may not be imposed on them and that their own wishes regarding end-of-life care will be honored.

In 2003, the Schiavo case was entering its final stages; arguments that had occupied the courts for 12 years—the soundness of the medical diagnosis, the possible self-interests of various parties, the credibility of witnesses, and so forth—seemed to have been exhausted or resolved. In April 2003, attorneys for Mary and Robert Schindler (Terri Schiavo's parents) made the extraordinary claim that "the wrong definitions were being applied to Ms. Schiavo."[38] The attorneys now claimed that Terri Schiavo should not be regarded as an individual in a dying state but as disabled. Not Dead Yet, along with 15 disability advocacy groups, filed an *amici curiae* brief on behalf of Mr. and Mrs. Schindler, based on their concern that the standards being applied to Terri Schiavo could be applied to "thousands of people with disabilities who, like Ms. Schiavo, cannot articulate their own views."[39]

Not long afterward, Not Dead Yet issued a news release charging that "disability issues are wrongly and misleadingly characterized as 'end-of-life' issues."[40] The target of its indignation was Last Acts, an end-of-life partnership supporting the development of palliative care initiatives for a wide range of patients with conditions such as Creutzfeldt-Jakob disease, Alzheimer's disease, amyotrophic lateral sclerosis, cerebral palsy, and multiple sclerosis.[41] The ideological wing of the disability rights movement regards palliative care as tantamount to neglect, viewing Last Acts and like organizations as perniciously attempting to subvert public perception of people with disabilities.[42] Steven Drake, research analyst for Not Dead Yet, accused end-of-life advocates of being the ones changing the frame, of attempting to mischaracterize or reframe what are properly aspects of "disability health care policy"—medically provided nutrition and hydration—as "end-of-life care."[43] The move here was to insist that patients who can be maintained on medically provided nutrition and hydration are not in fact dying. Were they to die, this view holds, it would be because they were "starved to death" and not as a result of underlying disease. According to Not Dead Yet, artificial nutrition and hydration should not be included in end-of-life policy "lest it become one."[44]

The proposed framing of Terri Schiavo as a disabled individual rather than a terminal patient or one in a permanent vegetative state—these words have obvious reference to well-known and widely accepted public policies in Florida—remapped the moral landscape in three ways. First, state statutes on end-of-life care would be rendered moot. Second, sympathy for Terri Schiavo could generate support for Not Dead Yet's ongoing campaign to challenge surrogate decision making via substituted judgment. Third, the apparent stakeholders would increase from the isolated and rare PVS patient and loved ones to include all who depend on others to effect their health care decisions (i.e., most hospice and nursing home patients and therefore, by extension, *everyone's* future self): "Terri Schiavo's fate is entwined with all disabled people who rely on surrogates."[45]

Max Lapertosa, attorney for the *amici*, challenged the idea that "terminating the life of a woman with severe disabilities" could be a "private family matter," insisting that the Schiavo case "reflects whether our society and legal system values the lives of people with disabilities equally to those without disabilities."[46] In these two sentences, disability rights advocates managed to associate the established end-of-life approach with humankind's most egregious historical injustices: Jim Crow laws and Nazi genocide. The cessation of medically provided nutrition and hydration was thus reframed as a human rights violation rather than a personal decision about medical care. As such, Terri Schiavo's actual wishes would have had no standing; she could not have consented to a violation of her human right (not to be deprived of life). Of course, this seems to conflict with human rights of self-sovereignty and bodily integrity; but, as we have seen, these rights have historically existed as male norms, i.e., male rights rather than human rights. Our discussion of gender supports the idea that rights of self-sovereignty and bodily integrity are either less tightly bound to the female (perhaps because they are more recent) or that they can be traded off for protection without the same sense of violation that might attach to such a tradeoff in the case of males, as the Miles and August study suggests.

In Schiavo, abortion foes joined the contingent of disability rights advocates in embracing the prolongation of medically provided nutrition and hydration, albeit from within competing frames. In part, this was possible because frames are fractional accounts of moral saliency and because both disability and anti-abortion advocates are "true believers" according to framing theory; that is, they were willing to discount or filter incorrigible evidence for the sake of maintaining their commitments. The Not Dead Yet alliance discounted Ms. Schiavo's expressed wishes. For his part, Governor Jeb Bush discounted his own staff's opinion that "Terri's Law," which authorized him to issue a one-time stay of the withdrawal of her tube, was unconstitutional, and in October 2003, he ordered her tube reinserted. In December 2003, in "true believer" fashion, Governor Bush shrugged off the report by Professor Jay Wolfson—whom the governor, himself, had selected as guardian *ad litem*—after Wolfson concluded that Ms. Schiavo was in a permanent vegetative state with no chance of improvement. In a letter released to the news media, the governor wrote:

> As I have said from the beginning, the state must protect every Floridian's right to life, and in so doing, err on the side of life. As Governor, I will continue to do just that. Nothing in Dr. Wolfson's report leads me to believe the stay should be lifted at this time, or that Mrs. Schiavo should be deprived of her right to live.[47]

:: The Fetal Protection Frame

The third reframing of the Schiavo case proceeded with the release by her parents of video clips from taped medical examinations: four minutes out of more than four hours of tape, showing the few times when Terri Schiavo's actions could be correlated with repeated entreaties to her. It was offered as a visual argument purporting to prove the Schindlers' contention that their daughter was not in a vegetative state and thus could not be denied nutrition and hydration, however administered; to do so would be to kill a sentient human, one who had a right to live, restricted though that life might be.

However, the video operates on deeper, more subliminal level. The images are reminiscent of the view through the "opaque womb"— Swedish photojournalist Lennart Nilsson's full-color portraits of an 18-week-old fetus published in *Life* magazine in 1965.

From this perspective, Theresa Schiavo is recast as a fully accessible fetus: she exhibits arousal without awareness, movement without intention; she is fully dependent on a specialized environment and relies on umbilical attachments—a PEG tube provides nutrition and hydration, and a catheter provides elimination.

The fetus image signifies vulnerability, helplessness, the need for protection. From Nilsson's fetal portraits to the anti-abortion propaganda video *The Silent Scream*[48] abortion foes have pursued a strategy of "making the fetus a public presence,"[49] a strategy well suited to a visual culture such as ours. The idea behind the public fetus strategy is that fetal images generate a visual bond, a form of recognition that will make abortion less likely.[50] With respect to the Schiavo video, that recognition response was amplified by virtue of the cumulative impact of public representations and of the ubiquitous *personal* representations of fetuses that abound given the routine use of obstetric ultrasound. The parade of politicians and elected representatives declaring Terri Schiavo to be sentient is a testament to the "conversion power of the [public] fetus."[51]

In addition to the emotional appeal that the fetal image evokes, the public fetus also serves as an abstract universal symbol of humanity and the right to life. Ultimately, the visual argument is not about Terri Schiavo; it is an argument by analogy against abortion *per se:* If one can be convinced to protect Terri Schiavo's life, despite the fact that she will never become aware, never outgrow her dependence on life support, never talk, love, feel, remember, or have any experience whatsoever;

then one cannot deny that same protection to vegetative-like humans, who are only *temporarily* dependent on life support (natural wombs), and who will come to self-consciousness.

:: Framing Women's Moral Agency

Frames are inevitably a partial account of the moral landscape. There are no "frame-free" perspectives. However, this does not render all perspectives equal: We can assess the validity and significance of what is included in—and what is excluded from—any given frame. All three of the Schiavo frames surveyed here reinforce culturally embedded views of women as moral patients rather than moral agents, as beings toward whom paternalism is appropriate, perhaps even obligatory.

In the gender frame, the prominent motif of the feminine is the opposite of agency: vacancy, passivity, and powerlessness. It is not only the unconscious, female patients who are represented as ineffectual: Mrs. Schindler, not Mr. Schindler, issues the call for rescuers to "save our baby;" Karen Quinlan's father was named her guardian, not her mother or both parents jointly.

In the disability rights frame, the motif of the feminine is efface-ment, subordination, and subservience. Political actors appropriate Terri Schiavo's narrative, her privacy, and her humanity in service of their agenda. Their frame shifts the focus of moral concern from Terri Schiavo's best interests as an individual to the interests of the collective she is obliged to represent—"the disabled."

The fetal frame is constructed to exclude the pregnant woman whose very body serves as life support. In *The Silent Scream*, the fetus hangs by its umbilicus, tethered to something invisible; fetal ultrasound photos seem to show the fetus in a tent-like habitat. In the Schiavo video, she occupies the entire screen; her mother is seen as a pair of hands reach-ing into the frame, an occasional glimpse of the back of someone's head. With the focus on Terri Schiavo, those appearances are unnoticeable.

Vitalism, the disproportionate valuation of mere life over other goods, informs both the disability rights frame and the fetal frame. It leads to its necessary conclusion—that life must always be preserved—only by obscuring the unceasing care that it entails and ignoring the humanity of those whose lives must fulfill the obligations of care. Notwithstanding the gender-neutral language, the caregiver is most likely to be a woman. The insistence on the unconditional protection of life is a grave insult to the agency and humanity of women.

Historically, social control of women has been maintained by enforcing gender norms, especially sexual and reproductive norms, effectively denying women morally significant forms of privacy and freedom that are essential to effective moral agency. While restrictions on abortion, contraception, and sexual orientation have epitomized the control of women through gender norms, autonomy must encompass choice in dying as well.

Analyses of women's continuing disadvantage despite formal guarantees of equality implicate the deep structure of our institutions, particularly the law and practices such as medicine that are significantly constituted by law and regulation. The dominant conceptions of equality, discrimination, and harm structure our thinking in such a way that important sources of women's disadvantage—external determination and stigma—cannot be apprehended as harms. What is needed is a commitment to improving our recognition of these dignitary harms in our policies and practices, and the resources to develop appropriate methods to do so.

The Schiavo discourse underscores the mutually reinforcing relationship between anti-abortion views and oppressive paternalism in end-of-life matters. Recognition of that relationship should cause us to be equally concerned about restrictions of autonomy in either context. While it is too early to say what impact the Schiavo case will have on these vast social issues, there is no doubt that it will be invoked incessantly and repeatedly to teach, to warn, to exhort, to challenge, and to extract meaning. There is indeed much to be learned from this case, and much to be learned from attention to gender.

NOTES TO CHAPTER 9

1. I am indebted to Jane Caputi, Hilde Lindemann, David G. Miller, and James Nelson for their valuable comments. Early versions of this paper were presented at the Florida Bioethics Network Conference (April 2004) and the American Society for Bioethics and the Humanities Sixth Annual Meeting (October 2004). I wish to acknowledge my colleagues in the Florida Bioethics Network for indispensable discussions, encouragement, and collaboration.

2. Jonas, H. Against the Stream: Comments on the definition of and redefinition of death. In T.L. Beauchamp and R.M. Veatch, eds. *Ethical Issues in Death and Dying*. Saddle River, N.J.: Prentice Hall, 1993, pp. 23–27 at p. 23. Jonas's essay was originally written in 1970 in response to the 1968 *Report of the Ad Hoc Committee of the Harvard Medical School to Examine*

the *Definition of Brain-death* (see *Journal of the American Medical Association* 1984;252:677–679), and it was first published in Jonas, H. *Philosophical Essays: From Ancient Creed to Technological Man.* Englewood Cliffs, N.J.: Prentice Hall, 1974.

3. As I use it here, "the Schiavo case" refers not to the protracted litigation but to the larger public debate. I distinguish between the central actor and the public discourse by using "Schiavo" to refer to the debate itself as an object of inquiry and "Terri Schiavo" to refer to her actual person. I have chosen not to refer to her by her first name alone to avoid either condescension or the false suggestion of personal familiarity. Both "Ms. Schiavo" (preferred by style editors) and "Mrs. Schiavo" avoid condescension but have the effect of submerging her person in a particular relationship.

4. Although legal arguments typically invoke neutral language, phrases such as "pregnant person" and male-normative concepts such as "reasonable person" or "rational" are understood to be gendered.

5. The concepts of "sex" and "gender" are complicated and contested, and are arguably more extensive than "male" and "female."

6. This applies as well to other social categories in which persisting attributes can be understood to have a kind of "acquired essentialism."

7. I adopt Hans Jonas's ("Against the Stream") way of speaking about the nature of the right in question. Similarly, in Miles, S., and August, A. Courts, Gender, and the "Right to Die." *Law, Medicine and Healthcare* 1990;18:85–95, Miles and August remind us that the "right to die" is properly described as "right to refuse life-sustaining treatment."

8. Gitlin, T. *The Whole World is Watching: Mass Media in the Making and Unmaking of the New Left (2d ed.).* Berkeley, Calif.: University of California Press, 2003 at p. 6.

9. Goffman, E. *Frame Analysis.* New York: Harper Row, 1974.

10. For a contrary view, see Kennedy, R. *Nigger—The Strange Career of a Troublesome Word.* New York: Pantheon, 2002.

11. Entman, R. Framing: Toward a clarification of a fractured paradigm. *Journal of Communication* 1993;43(4):51–58.

12. Lakoff, G. *Framing: It's About Values and Ideas.* Rockridge Institute, 2006. Available at http://www.rockridgeinstitute.org/research/lakoff/valuesideas

13. Entman, "Framing: Toward a clarification."

14. Anderson, I.D. *The Role of Framing in Public Policy Debate: An Experimental Research Design.* Working Paper #384. Presented at the Midwest Political Science Association Annual Meeting in Chicago, Illinois, April 27–30, 2000. HTML-only version available at http://ascc.artsci.wustl.edu/~polisci/papers/andersona.html.

15. Tisch, C. High profile cases share characteristic (Interview with Steven Miles, MD, Center for Bioethics, University of Minnesota). *St. Petersburg Times,* March 18, 2005. Available at http://www.sptimes.com/2005/03/18/Tampabay/Postcards_offend_some.shtml.

16. Yount, L. *Physician Assisted Suicide and Euthanasia.* New York: Facts on File, Inc., 2000.

17. Raymond, D. 'Fatal Practices': A feminist analysis of physician-assisted suicide and euthanasia. *Hypatia* 1999;14(2):1–25.

18. Ibid.

19. Davis, D.S. Why suicide is like contraception. In M.P. Battin, R. Rhodes, and A. Silvers, eds. *Feminism and Bioethics: Beyond Reproduction*. New York: Oxford University Press, 1996.

20. Wolf, S.M. Gender, Feminism, and Death: Physician-assisted suicide and euthanasia. In S.M. Wolf. *Feminism and Bioethics: Beyond Reproduction*. New York: Oxford University Press, 1996.

21. Miles and August, "Courts, Gender."

22. Ibid.

23. Miles and August (ibid.) do consider whether men's constructed preferences for refusing life support are too easily accepted in virtue of the aforementioned views about medical technology and masculine agency, but conclude that men are protected by the fact that their families "bear their preferences to court" and would not concur unless they believed that such care was unwanted or not in the patient's best interest.

24. See a variety of responses to Steven Mile's interview with Tisch, "High Profile Cases" on *Alas! A blog*. Available at http://www.amptoons.com/blog/archives/2005/03/25/is-it-because-terris-a-girl.

25. Didion, J. The case of Theresa Schiavo. *The New York Review of Books* June 9, 2005;52:1–17 at p. 14.

26. I thank Jane Caputi for suggesting this point.

27. Wolf, S.M. Nancy Beth Cruzan: No voice at all. *Hastings Center Report* 1990;20(1):38–41 at p. 40.

28. See, for example, Morgan, S. *Into Our Own Hands: The Women's Health Movement in the United States 1969–1990*. N.J.: Rutgers University Press, 2002. See also Sherwin, S. *No Longer Patient: Feminist Ethics and Health Care*. Philadelphia: Temple University Press, 1992.

29. Partnership for Caring. *Women and End-of-Life Decisions*. Washington, D.C.: Partnership for Caring, 2001. For further information, see: American College of Obstetricians and Gynecologists. End-of-life decision making. In *Ethics in Obstetrics and Gynecology*, 2nd ed. Washington, D.C.: American College of Obstetrics and Gynecology, 2004. Available at http://www.acog.org/from_home/publications/ethics/ethics060.pdf. See also, Stoll, K.D. *Pregnancy Exclusions in State Living Will and Medical Proxy Statutes*. Washington, D.C.: The Center for Women Policy Studies, 1992. Available at http://www.centerwomenpolicy.org/pdfs/RRH1.pdf. For an updated list of legislation in this area, sorted by state, see http://estate.findlaw.com/estate-planning/living-wills/estate-planning-law-state-living-wills.html.

30. The historical precedents include court-ordered cesarean delivery, appointment of guardian *ad litem* for fetuses, and prosecution of pregnant women who test positive for illegal substances, do not follow doctor's recommendations, or fail to keep prenatal appointments.

31. Rothberg, K.H. Feminism, law and bioethics. *Kennedy Institute of Ethics Journal* 1996;6(1):69–84.

32. Rosser, S.V. *Women's Health: Missing from United States Medicine.* Bloomington, Ind.: Indiana University Press, 1994.
33. See http://www.nrlc.org/euthanasia/SandD/index.html. For an analysis by Florida bioethicists of the "Model Starvation and Dehydration of Persons with Disabilities Prevention Act" in its Florida version (HB701), see Florida Bioethics Leaders' Commentary on HB701, March 7, 2005, Corrected 3–10. Available at the March 7, 2005, Timeline entry at http://www.miami.edu/ethics/schiavo/schiavo_timeline.html. HB701 is available under the entry for February 18, 2005.
34. Garret, J., Harris, R., Norbum, J., Patrick, D., and Danis, M. Life-sustaining treatments during terminal illness: who wants what? *Journal of General Internal Medicine* 1993;8(July):361–368.
35. For discussion of this issue, see Dresser R. Schiavo's Legacy: the need for an objective standard. *Hastings Center Report* 2005;35(June/July)(3): 20–22.
36. Art. I, sec. 23.
37. *In Re Browning*, 568 So. 2d 4 (Fla. 1990).
38. Cooper-Dowda, R. Pay No Attention to the Woman Behind the Curtain!!!!: Attending Terri Schiavo's appeals hearing on April 4, 2003. Not Dead Yet, April 4, 2003. Available at http://www.notdeadyet.org/docs/schiavoupdateapr403.html.
39. Not Dead Yet. National Disability Groups Outraged about "End of Life" Advocacy further Devaluing Life with a Disability. Not Dead Yet press release, June 23, 2003. Available at http://notdeadyet.org/docs/lastactspr.html.
40. Ibid.
41. Last Acts, which ceased its activities in 2005, was a national coalition of partners—including the American Medical Association, the American Cancer Society, and many other health care, bioethics, religious, and consumer groups—funded by the Robert Wood Johnson Foundation and the Partnership for Caring. Its aim was to improve care and caring near the end of life through information gathering/data sharing, and public awareness initiatives on death-related issues. Following a public event that included a one-sided discussion of the Robert Wendland case, Not Dead Yet charged Last Acts with trying to set health care policy for people with disabilities while excluding disability advocate groups from the process. For Not Dead Yet's charges, see http://www.notdeadyet.org/docs/lastactsflyer.html and http://www.notdeadyet.org/docs/responsetolastacts.html.
42. There are many disability advocacy organizations and not all share the positions of Not Dead Yet. AUTONOMY (http://www.autonomynow.org) is a disability rights advocacy organization based in Massachusetts that represents the interest of "persons with disabilities who expect choice in all aspects of their lives, including choice at the end of life." Other prominent disability organizations such as the Brain Injury Association of America, the Christopher Reeve Paralysis Foundation, the Parkinson's Action Network, and the ALS Association did not take positions on Schiavo. See Connolly, C. Schiavo raised profile of disabled. *Washington Post*, April 2, 2005. Available at http://www.washingtonpost.com.

43. Drake, S. Changing the words, reframing the issue: a brief history. *Ragged Edge Online*, July 21, 2003. Available at http://www.raggededgemagazine.com/extra/drake/071203.html.

44. Although the characterization of medically provided nutrition and hydration as a "treatment" that may be refused has been settled at law, increased activity by disability rights activists and Pope John Paul II's March 20, 2004, address to the World Federation of Catholic Medical Associations and Pontifical Academy for Life Congress on "Life-Sustaining Treatments and Vegetative State: Scientific Advances and Ethical Dilemmas" (available at http://www.vatican.va/holy_father/john_paul_ii/speeches/2004/march/documents/hf_jp-ii_spe_20040320_congress-fiamc_en.html) have had an unsettling impact on legislators, residents, and health care providers in Florida, and no doubt elsewhere as well.

45. Disability Rights Watch. Issues surrounding Terri Schindler-Schiavo are disability rights issues, say national disability organizations. *Disability Rights Watch*, October 27, 2003. Available at http://www.zmag.org/disabilityrights.htm.

46. Not Dead Yet, "Disability Groups."

47. Bush, J. Statement by Governor Jeb Bush [on] guardian *ad litem's* report, December 2, 2003. Available at http://sun6.dms.state.fl.us/eog_new/eog/library/releases/2003/December/litems-report_12-2-03.html

48. *The Silent Scream* (American Portrait Films, 1984) purports to show the termination of a 12-week-fetus in which the fetus attempts to elude the surgical instrument and utters an open-mouthed scream that is interpreted for viewers as "pain." It was actually a series of still ultrasound images, not a video recording; the apparent "scream" was accomplished via camera sleight of hand, aided by dramatic auditory cues and an authoritative voice over. It was not even an accurate "re-enactment" of such a procedure; movement at that stage could only have been reflexive, not intentional, and the cognitive development is insufficient for pain sensation. The preceding synopsis of the film is based on Petchesky, R.P. Fetal images: the power of visual culture in the politics of reproduction. *Feminist Studies* 1987;13:263–292.

49. In this section, I adapt Rosalind Petchesky's analysis of fetal imagery in *The Silent Scream* to develop points about the Schiavo video. See Petchesky, R.P. *Abortion and Women's Choice: The State, Sexuality, and Reproductive Freedom*. Boston: Northeastern University Press, 1990.

50. Petchesky, "Abortion and Women's Choice," locates the source of the visual bonding strategy in Fletcher, J.C. and Evans M.I. Maternal bonding in early fetal ultrasound examinations. *New England Journal of Medicine* 1983;308:392–393, in which the authors claim that ultrasound images may make it more likely that "ambivalent pregnancies" will be "resolved in favor of the fetus."

51. Ginsburg, F. *Contested Lives: The Abortion Debate in an American Community*. Berkeley: University of California Press, 1989. Quoted in Taylor, J.S. The public foetus and the family car: from abortion politics to a Volvo advertisement. *Science as Culture* 1993;3/4:601–618.

10 ::

Terri Schiavo and Televised News:
Fact or Fiction?

Robert M. Walker
Jay Black

In the early years of the Terri Schiavo case, there was little to distinguish it from earlier cases that had made their way into courts across the country. The issue of tube feeding patients in a persistent vegetative state (PVS) had already been addressed by a number of state courts, including Florida's Supreme Court.[1] The tube feeding issue was also at the center of the U.S. Supreme Court case involving Nancy Cruzan.[2] Indeed, the Schiavo case mirrored the Cruzan case in many respects. Both cases involved young married women who suffered anoxic encephalopathy; both were left in a PVS; neither had an advance directive; and both cases involved deciding whether to discontinue tube feeding. In addition, both women came from Catholic families, and both had parents who were actively involved in their legal cases. The only difference seems to have been that Nancy Cruzan's parents fought to have their daughter's feeding tube removed, while Terri Schiavo's parents struggled to keep their daughter's tube in place.

:: A Media-Friendly Case

Despite having little to set it apart ethically and legally from earlier cases, the Schiavo case nevertheless became the most publicized tube feeding case in American jurisprudence. Several features of the case made it particularly attractive to televised news media. The most obvious feature was the intense and unprecedented family conflict. In seeking to have Ms. Schiavo's feeding tube removed, her husband, Michael, claimed he wanted only to honor his wife's wishes, while her parents, Robert and Mary Schindler, were convinced their daughter would never choose to starve to death. The conflict was complicated by unsavory accusations on both sides as well as unparalleled legal rancor. So intense was the legal fight that Ms. Schiavo's guardian *ad litem* referred to it as "nearly ten years of legal hostilities" characterized by a series of "extensive, extraordinary, exquisite, nearly acrobatic legal efforts."[3]

A second media-friendly feature of the case was the unusual willingness of Ms. Schiavo's parents, particularly her father, to use television to put forward their point of view. In previous cases, families seemed to have avoided the media entirely, or at least shied away from attention. Ms. Schiavo's father, on the other hand, appeared to embrace TV news as a tool to further his fight to save his daughter. He was frequently interviewed on news broadcasts and apparently grew quite comfortable on camera.

The third and most influential feature accounting for the unusual media attention given to the case was the widespread availability of video that showed Ms. Schiavo blinking, moving, and making facial expressions. No other PVS case in history has had as much visual material or exposure. When video of Ms. Schiavo was accompanied by her father's comment that she could respond to those around her, many people found it easy to agree with him. Seeing is believing. The apparent harmony of images and words put on the defensive anyone who would suggest that things were not as they seemed. This also created a natural suspicion of Ms. Schiavo's husband, who remained silent, choosing to speak almost entirely through his attorney. Many viewers doubted his motives and sincerity, seeing him as inexplicably bent on denying his wife treatment and even basic food and water.

The result of this extraordinary media exposure, especially on television news programs, was to generate great public interest in the case and create political pressure on Florida's lawmakers and governor to intervene. In the days following the removal of Ms. Schiavo's feeding tube in October 2003, the pressure on lawmakers became so intense that the Florida Legislature passed a hastily drafted law authorizing the governor to set aside the court's decision and order a surgical procedure that would provide her with a new feeding tube.[4] Ms. Schiavo's parents, it seemed, had finally won a victory. Having lost time and again in the courts of law, they won by taking their daughter's case to the media and to the court of public opinion.

∷ The Mandates of TV News

But did the public perception of this case, mediated via television, reflect the truth, or did the media, by their very nature, distort key issues in the case and thereby create a false impression? Why did there seem to be significant differences between the "reality" of the Schiavo case as played out on television and as played out in the courts?

Consider the basic nature of television coverage. According to veteran journalist Robert MacNeil, the unfortunate operating mandate behind televised news "is to keep everything brief, not to strain the attention of anyone but instead to provide constant stimulation through variety, novelty, action, and movement. You are required . . . to pay attention to no concept, no character, and no problem for more than a few seconds at a time." The controlling assumptions are that "bite-sized is best, that complexity must be avoided, that nuances are dispensable, that qualifications impede the simple message, that visual stimulation is a substitute for thought, and that verbal precision is an anachronism."[5]

Events, rather than underlying issues, dominate television news, and predictable events—what historian Daniel Boorstin called "pseudo-events"[6]—such as press conferences or protests stand the greatest chance of being covered. This is not only because assignment editors can plan how to allocate their camera crews and reporters, but also because such events are easy to cover, with their predictable visual images and sound bites. Veteran lobbyists and special pleaders know how to play to television's attraction for the predictable, the visual, and the dramatic. They know not to violate television's Eleventh Commandment: "Thou shalt not bore." As MacNeil said, "All television gravitates towards drama, and what passes for drama is often belligerence, people barking at each other, like soap opera actors, sounding vehement to make up for cardboard characters or too little rehearsal time."[7]

These verities of television news are neither amoral nor accidental. They are, at best, non-moral craft-based variables. They result from an unwritten agreement between commercial television and its viewers, aided, of course, by well-paid consultants who tell broadcasters how to package the day's real events and pseudo-events to deliver the largest number of eyeballs to the advertisers. Viewer preferences drive mainstream coverage. Their votes, whether cast by their remote controls or Nielsen ratings—or delivered by consultants—tell news producers what stories to cover, how to cover them, even what the reporters and anchors and news sets should look like. (Hint: When the furniture on the set gets rearranged or the anchor sports a new hairstyle, the show is in ratings trouble.)

In summarizing how temporal, spatial, technological, and judgmental factors affect television news, critics Mankiewicz and Swerdlow have described some of the informal and unacknowledged laws of television news:

> Unattractive faces are almost never on camera in "good guy" roles; a fire at night will almost always be shown though an equally serious daytime fire won't; every news story must be complete within one minute and fifteen seconds, unless the program is doing an "in-depth" treatment, in which case one minute and forty-five seconds may be permitted. All this has led to an overriding law—The Trivial Will Always Drive Out the Serious. There are other limitations and strictures. A story with film, for example, will almost always take precedence over one that must be read from the anchor desk or reported in a "stand-up" on the spot. If there is film, the action film will almost always replace the film that includes only a conversation or a discussion—"talking heads" are to be avoided if at all possible.[8]

Although Mankiewicz and Swerdlow's critique was written nearly a generation ago, it still rings disturbingly true, except that today a 1-minute-and-45-second news story is referred to as a "documentary."

What do these rules of television mean to the viewer? Does television's preference for the visual mean broadcast news is geared to the emotional rather than the intellectual? Does the emphasis on action rather than thought, events rather than concepts, conflicts rather than underlying issues, mean television news is devoid of explanation and nuance and is, therefore, comprehensible only to the already well-informed members of the public? Is it possible that most television news reporting does little, if anything, to develop audiences' potential to analyze, think independently, or learn from grasping social patterns in the unfolding of events?

Contrast the controlling ideas of television news with the controlling ideas of jurisprudence. In legal cases, judges have no interest in catering to short attention spans, nor are they concerned with keeping anyone stimulated through novelty and variety. While television abhors dwelling on a concept or topic for more than a moment, the courts will painstakingly explore concepts, problems, and questions of fact for as long as may be required. Unlike television's approach, complexity in legal cases must be grappled with; nuances are not only important, but indispensable; qualifications and explanations are not impediments, but the very points upon which issues of life and death turn. There is no simple message to convey; instead, there is concern for truth and correct judgment. Verbal precision, far from being abandoned as anachronistic, is the cornerstone of clear understanding.

:: The Bias of Objectivity

To a journalist, objectivity is an institutional craft value advocating impartiality or fairness, or stressing impersonal detachment. Whether "myth" or "standard operating procedure," objectivity has had a long shelf life in media criticism.[9] The Schiavo coverage is a case in point.

The mantra of many a newscast (and the slogan, by the way, of Fox News) is that its coverage is "fair and balanced." The implication is that fair and balanced coverage will also be objective coverage. However, the media's requirements for fair and balanced coverage are often greatly simplified. To be "fair," a reporter need only give time to both sides. To be "balanced," the reporter need only give both sides equal time. To be "objective," the reporter must avoid passing judgment, but instead keep everything controversial and open to question. Through these techniques reporters not only create the impression of unbiased reporting, they also extend the story's potential impact and life, since a story without controversy can hardly be expected to capture and hold the attention of viewers.

Journalism professor Michael Ryan says objectivity has gotten a bad rap, that the debate has been one-sided because of definitional flaws. Ryan argues that media and society would be better served if journalists practiced the same type of objectivity employed by thoughtful scientists, using analytical and interpretive skills in collecting and disseminating information that describes multifaceted reality as accurately as possible; refusing to support any political, social, economic, or cultural interests; seeking the most informed, qualified, forthcoming sources available to address the many sides of issues; helping audiences decide which truth claims are the most compelling; being individually and institutionally accountable.[10]

However, as sociologists Gaye Tuchman and Herbert Gans explained in their groundbreaking studies of journalists in the 1970s, the ideal and the real don't always mesh. Tuchman's classic introduction to the conflict maintained that journalists must make immediate decisions concerning validity, reliability, and truth in order to address the problems imposed by the nature of processing news, which she said "leaves no time for reflexive epistemological examination."[11] She said journalists struggle to identify and verify facts and truth-claims, and that problems arise for news audiences when unverifiable truth claims—particularly those by "experts"—are paired or left unadorned in the daily news. Journalists mislead themselves about their own objectivity when they make heavy use of opinions and quotes from sources; reporters falsely believe they are "removing themselves from participation in the story."[12]

Gans, in a study of major national news media, said that in selecting stories to cover and the methods to be used, journalists "strive to be objective, both in intent, by applying personal detachment; and in effect, by disregarding the implications of the news."[13] However, Gans demonstrated that despite journalists' proclamations of detachment and objectivity, their work products clearly display a pattern of enduring values, unconsciously and implicitly valuing ethnocentrism, altruistic democracy, responsible capitalism, small-town pastoralism, individualism, "moderatism," social order, and national leadership.[14]

The challenges of being an objective journalist are morally significant. Recently several arguments have been raised asking for a revised definition of the term, a "softening" of expectations about whether or how journalists can be objective. Michael Ryan has said journalists in a democracy have a "moral covenant" with their audiences to provide "complete, balanced, fair, and accurate information and commentary." Admitting that "pure objectivity" is unattainable, he advocated an "objective approach" that would find journalists attempting to provide information that is complete, precise, balanced, and accurate; viewing powerful authorities and institutions with skepticism; considering new evidence and alternative interpretations; serving no religious, economic, social, or political agendas; recognizing their own predispositions and not allowing those predispositions to determine outcomes; using creativity in the search for facts and opinions that don't conform to the dominant narrative; and sharing all information freely.[15]

Jay Rosen, recognized as the intellectual founder of the "public journalism" movement, has noted that:

> Objectivity can mean many things in journalism. The disinterested pursuit of truth, the care to ground reporting in verifiable facts, the principled attempt to restrain one's own biases and avoid prejudice are core values from which the press draws practical guidance and moral strength. No one should trifle with them. But objectivity also has its weaknesses. Under its

influence "facts" tend to be placed in one category, "opinions" or personal views in another; with this division the journalist's mind appears to be successfully mapped. This works for some purposes . . . but there is a whole category of intellectual work that eludes the language of objectivity, with its attendant concerns about "bias."[16]

Whether there are objectively occurring events is not the issue; the debate is over whether news can be an objective enterprise. Cole Campbell, former editor of the *St. Louis Post-Dispatch,* said, "It's absolutely correct to say that there are objectively occurring events . . . Speeches are made, volcanoes erupt, trees fall. But," he continued, *"news is not a scientifically observable event. News is a choice, an extraction process, saying that one event is more meaningful than another event. The very act of saying that means making judgments that are based on values and based on frames."*[17]

With these distinctions in mind, we can turn to some of the other "biases" that governed television coverage of the Terri Schiavo case.

:: The Bias of Perceived Credibility

In televised news reports on the Schiavo case, it was common to see stories equally covering both points of view—that of Ms. Schiavo's husband and that of her parents. Yet despite this apparent balance, the potential for bias remains. The first area of potential bias concerns the issue of apparent credibility. In televised news media, one's credibility depends not on one's education, expertise, and knowledge, but on how well one comes across on camera. According to communications theorist Neal Postman,

> The credibility of the teller is the ultimate test of the truth of a proposition. "Credibility" here does not refer to the past record of the teller for making statements that have survived the rigors of reality-testing. It refers only to the impression of sincerity, authenticity, vulnerability or attractiveness (choose one or more) conveyed by the actor/reporter.[18]

In televised reports on the case, Ms. Schiavo's father clearly came across as more credible. He was comfortable on camera and spoke with an appealing sincerity. Her husband, on the other hand, chose to let his attorney speak for him. His discomfort on camera and his personal silence left many viewers cold and gave them the impression that he had something to hide. His explanation for not engaging in interviews was that he never sought to publicize his wife's situation, but instead tried to maintain her privacy. Even so, the result was that most viewers readily identified with Ms. Schiavo's father and found him more believable. So despite equal time being given to both sides, the credibility gap led to a bias in favor of her father.[19]

Consider the images of other protagonists and newsmakers in the Schiavo saga: Randall Terry, who founded the anti-abortion group "Operation Rescue"; Florida Governor Jeb Bush (who rushed "Terri's Law" through the legislature and was, for all intents and purposes, sincere in his right-to-life stance) and his brother, President George W. Bush (who rushed back to Washington, D.C., from his Texas vacation to petition Congress to redress his grievances); the Rev. Jesse Jackson (who aligned himself with the religious right); Senator/physician William Frist (who viewed the controversial videotape and concluded that Ms. Schiavo was not in a PVS); the Pope; an endless array of attorneys and judges; and random protesters. The credibility meter, despite journalists' futile attempts to "balance" the presentations, was tilted in favor of the most articulate, the most passionate, the most photogenic. Such is the nature of news.

:: The Bias of Open Questions

Another area of potential bias concerns the matter of truthfulness or fidelity to established facts. Journalists, as noted above, deal with truth claims and are responsible for balancing them according to unwritten standards of veracity and significance. Not many journalists grapple philosophically with issues of epistemology, but all of them try hard to avoid passing along blatant untruths. It is more than a simple matter of terminology; it is a matter of first principles.

The tendency in televised news is to depart from epistemological inquiry in order to keep the story controversial and alive. The central technique involves presenting established facts as if they are open to question. For example, it was common to see televised reports on the Schiavo case cast doubt upon the PVS diagnosis. Long after the matter of her diagnosis had been settled, reporters continued saying that Ms. Schiavo was in "what some doctors call a persistent vegetative state." In making these kinds of attributions, reporters repeatedly gave the impression that there was real controversy over the diagnosis, and that only some doctors thought she was in a PVS. When this statement was coupled with video of Ms. Schiavo, and her father's flat denial that his daughter was in a PVS, viewers were led to believe that there was real doubt about the diagnosis.

The truth was that the diagnosis was firmly established. Several qualified physicians and specialists had examined and tested Ms. Schiavo. All but two concluded that she was in a PVS. Virtually unreported was the fact that these two physicians were offering their unproven and proprietary treatments; thus, they had a significant conflict of interest. The courts, after weighing the evidence and assessing the validity and credibility of the medical testimony, consistently concluded that Ms. Schiavo was in a PVS. Even the independent guardian appointed by Governor Bush conducted a careful review and concluded that she was in a PVS and that the evidence was compelling.[20] Nevertheless, television news reporters repeatedly presented the matter of the diagnosis as if it were a point of great controversy. Another important example of forsaking fact for the sake of story involved the matter of treatment for Ms. Schiavo. While news reporters frequently mentioned that treatment for her PVS had been offered by two of the physicians involved in her case, the reporters made no judgment about whether the proposed treatments were legitimate or not. What the reporters left unstated was that the two treatments in question, vasodilation therapy and hyperbaric therapy, had been thoroughly considered by the trial court. The court found a "total absence of supporting case studies or medical literature" that would support the use of either vasodilation therapy or hyperbaric therapy in patients in a PVS.[21] In addition, any proposed treatment would have to do the impossible, namely regrow or recreate the missing parts of Ms. Schiavo's brain. It was almost never reported that most of her cerebral cortex, the part of the brain that thinks, feels, and perceives, was destroyed more than a decade earlier when she suffered a cardiac arrest and stopped breathing.

By not reporting the facts about the proposed treatments, a reporter maintains the veneer of objectivity by not taking sides. This nevertheless leaves the viewer with the clear and erroneous impression that Ms. Schiavo was being denied treatment for her condition. When her father ratified that impression on many occasions by saying that his daughter was being denied treatment, viewers were left to think that a terrible injustice was taking place, that treatment that could help her was being withheld. In reality, the fact that her condition was untreatable was a settled matter. Presenting it as an open issue was not only unfaithful to the facts; it deceived viewers and did much injustice to Terri Schiavo.

Another basic semantic and epistemological problem throughout the coverage of the case was journalists' seeming inability to strike a balance between "objective" medical science and "subjective" moral beliefs. As researchers have noted,

> Some journalists used terms such as "right to live" and "right to die" or "extending her life" and "prolonging her death" interchangeably. Some casually repeated pejoratively inaccurate words such as "murder" and "starvation." Some printed or uttered value-laden phrases such as "saving her life" and "Terri's champions" indiscriminately.[22]

There is no doubt that this was a particularly difficult environment for journalists to gather and report firmly established facts and truth. General assignment reporters—many of whom were parachuted into St. Petersburg ill prepared for the complex situation—had to produce, on deadline, news accounts that advanced the story. Even local reporters, who had lived for 14 years with the story and knew the local players, were overwhelmed by the carnival of competing claims. Little wonder there was a tendency to ask "open questions."

:: The Bias of Visual Emphasis

A final source of bias in televised news stories resulted from reporters selecting only those aspects of the case that could be effectively presented visually, punctuated by sound bites. This meant that critical issues might have been underreported because they wouldn't play well on television. A good example is the issue of Ms. Schiavo's wishes. Because there is no video of her expressing her wishes, and no sound bites from relatives who remember her past statements, the matter of Ms. Schiavo's end-of-life wishes was downplayed in the media and therefore in the minds of viewers.

The courts, on the other hand, had carefully addressed the issue of her wishes, having heard testimony from both sides. The courts heard testimony from relatives and friends regarding her past statements on treatment at the end of life. Of the statements given, a number were recent statements made by a mature Terri Schiavo on serious occasions such as funerals or times when a loved one was seriously ill. These statements, recalled by her husband and a couple of her in-laws, whom she had grown close to, all indicated that Ms. Schiavo would not choose to remain on artificial nutrition and hydration in the devastating setting of a PVS. On the other side, her parents said they believed she would want to be kept alive, based on a statement she made when she was a young girl hearing about the Karen Quinlan case. A high school friend also testified that her reaction to the Karen Quinlan case appeared to remain consistent into her high school years. The testimony about Ms. Schiavo's earlier statements seemed to reflect a sentiment toward continuing treatment, especially when there is some uncertainty about the outcome.

The judge regarded the more recent, mature, and serious statements as having greater weight than statements made before adulthood. He also found the more recent statements to be sufficiently clear and convincing as to warrant the conclusion that Ms. Schiavo would not want to be maintained in a PVS on a feeding tube. By contrast, the televised news media, in failing to report the court's examination of Ms. Schiavo's wishes, continually left viewers with the impression that she had no opinion about how she would want to be cared for. This is certainly a vital point, for if those viewers supporting the parents and governor had been made aware that she wouldn't have wanted the feeding tube, they might very well have arrived at a different opinion on the central issue in the case.

Much of this was too nuanced for television's vast visual maw. Lacking recent video of Ms. Schiavo (courts had forbidden either the Schindlers' or Michael Schiavo's advocates—or anyone else—from taking still or video pictures of her in the nursing home), television had to use old images, pictures of courthouse doors, or the current day's protesters. The oft-viewed and oft-maligned tape made years earlier by Ms. Schiavo's parents seemed to show her to be capable of thought, speech, and the ability to communicate. However, as bioethicist Art Caplan describes it, it was a heavily edited piece of advocacy, excerpts culled from hours and hours of taping. "Family members would move into Terri's field of vision to make it look like she was 'looking' at them. Her grimaces and twitches were edited to appear as smiles."[23] Caplan said that television simply could not resist showing the tape, running it round the clock as though it were a documentary—in the process doing more "to undermine the public's understanding of what it means for a person to be in a permanent vegetative state than any single piece of video ever broadcast in the United States."[24] That tape, of course, also influenced politicians (Jeb and George Bush, Senator Frist, and others) and muddled public policy decisions.

Toward the end, the vigil outside the Woodside Hospice had become a media circus, created for and eagerly devoured by television cameras and reporters. Moments after Terri Schiavo's death, a man began to play his trumpet, and he was immediately surrounded by a gaggle of cameramen, two or three deep.[25] As described by *St. Petersburg Times* TV columnist Chase Squires, TV news outlets had plenty of images to help tell the story of Ms. Schiavo's death, even though most of them—of the tearful family members, talkative advocates and protesters with signs, shrines and flowers—supported Mrs. Schiavo's parents:

> What viewers saw, as TV delivered what it could live and largely unedited, was a blur of hastily convened news conferences, protesters and political sound bites. There even were aerial shots eerily reminiscent of the O. J. Simpson chase as news helicopters followed the white van carrying Mrs. Schiavo's body to the Medical Examiner's Office.[26]

Television is a visual medium. The medium lives by its ratings, by its capacity to deliver viewers to advertisers. To curse it for presenting dramatic, gripping images at the expense of thoughtful analysis is overly simplistic. On the other hand, to ask it somehow to dampen the feeding frenzy and provide perspective is fully justified. Even veteran reporters who were fully immersed in the Schiavo coverage now say they wish they had had the individual and institutional support to pull back occasionally and provide the bigger picture. Mark Douglas, of WFLA-TV in Tampa, said he "felt like a pebble tossed by a tumbling wave, swept to a place not of my choosing."[27]

▪▪ The TV News Portrayal of the Case

The Terri Schiavo case is the most highly publicized tube feeding case ever. It attracted unprecedented media attention, not because of questions of law or ethics, but because it was a compelling story full of conflict, accusations, debatable diagnoses, denied treatments, and the dramatic and incredible intervention by Florida's Legislature and governor. It was also compelling because at its center was a father fighting for the life of his daughter against the system, which seemed determined to force her death through dehydration and starvation. Yet much of this was hyperbole, frenzy, and spin—all put forward for the sake of keeping the story alive.

But what of Terri Schiavo? Would she have wanted to be kept alive as she was? The second District Court of Appeal cut through the smokescreen and rightly identified her right to decide as the central issue in this case: "But in the end this case is not about the aspirations that loving parents have for their children. It is about Theresa Schiavo's right to make her own decision, independent of her parents and independent of her husband."[28]

In overlooking this, the media have played a key role in frustrating Ms. Schiavo's right to be free of unwanted medical intervention. Though the reporting was in many cases fair, balanced, and objective by media standards—and may very well have helped many people understand end-of-life issues and the need for living wills—it paradoxically left viewers with the false impressions that Ms. Schiavo might not have been in a PVS, that she might have improved if she were not denied treatment, and that nothing was known of her wishes. The media's treatment of the case, while perhaps improving ratings for its news shows, did not improve her situation, nor did it adequately educate the public. Instead, the result was to agitate and inflame public sentiment about the case, based not on truth and fact, but on misimpressions largely fueled by the televised news media's misleading portrayal.

Shortly after the death of Terri Schiavo, the American public was treated to an award-winning film about some of television's finest hours, its courageous coverage of Senator Joseph McCarthy. In that film (*Good Night, and Good Luck*) newsman Edward R. Murrow described the paradox of television, a paradox that has most certainly come to light in television's coverage of the Terri Schiavo case. In a 1958 speech to the Radio Television News Directors Association, Murrow observed that:

> This instrument can teach, it can illuminate; yes, and it can even inspire. But it can do so only to the extent that humans are determined to use it to those ends. Otherwise it is merely wires and lights in a box. There is a great and perhaps decisive battle to be fought against ignorance, intolerance, and indifference. This weapon of television could be useful.[29]

NOTES TO CHAPTER 10

1. *In re Browning*, 568 So. 2d 4 (Fla. 1990).
2. *Cruzan v Director, Missouri Department of Health*, 110 S Ct 2841 (1990).
3. Wolfson, J., Guardian *Ad Litem* for Theresa Marie Schiavo. *Report to Governor Jeb Bush and the 6th Judicial Circuit in the Matter of Theresa Marie Schiavo* (Dec. 1, 2003) at p. 35. Available under the Timeline entry for December 1, 2003, at http://www.miami.edu/ethics/schiavo/schiavo_ timeline.html.
4. Chapter 2003–418, Laws of Florida (popularly known as "Terri's Law").

5. Robert MacNeil quoted in Postman, N. *Amusing Ourselves to Death: Public Discourse in the Age of Show Business*. New York: Penguin Books, 1985, at p. 105.
6. Boorstin, D. *The Image: A Guide to Pseudo-events in America*. New York: Harper & Row, Harper Colophon Books, 1964.
7. MacNeil, R. *The Mass Media and Public Trust*: Occasional Paper, No. 1. New York: Gannett Center for Media Studies, 1985.
8. Mankiewicz, F., and Swerdlow, J. *Remote Control: Television and the Manipulation of American Life*. New York: Ballantine Books, 1978, 97–98.
9. The term "objectivity" may have created a semantic divide between journalists and philosophers; the latter use the term "objectivism" to describe doctrines that stress the objective reality of what is known or perceived. The differences may give rise to significant debates between the media and philosophy communities.
10. Ryan, M. Journalistic ethics, objectivity, existential journalism, standpoint epistemology, and public journalism. *Journal of Mass Media Ethics* 2001;16(1): 3–5.
11. Tuchman, G. Objectivity as strategic ritual: An examination of newsmen's notions of objectivity. *American Journal of Sociology* 1972;77(4): 660–679 at p. 662.
12. Ibid., p. 668.
13. Gans, H.J. *Deciding What's News: A study of CBS Evening News, NBC Nightly News, Newsweek and Time*. New York: Vintage Books, 1980, p. 183.
14. Ibid. at pp. 42–69.
15. Ryan, M. Mainstream news media, an objective approach, and the march to war in Iraq. *Journal of Mass Media Ethics* 2006;21(1):4–29.
16. Rosen, J. *Getting the Connections Right: Public Journalism and the Troubles in the Press*. New York: The Twentieth Century Fund Press, 1996, p. 29.
17. Cole Campbell quoted in James Fallows, *Breaking the News: How the Media Undermine American Democracy*. New York: Pantheon, 1996, p. 262.
18. Postman, *Amusing Ourselves*, p. 102.
19. Douglas, M. Commentary 1: Duke Righteous meets Terri Schiavo. *Journal of Mass Media Ethics* 2006;21(2&3):217–219.
20. Wolfson, *Report*, p. 33.
21. *In re Schiavo*, 90–2908GB-003 (Fla Cir Ct, Pinellas Co, 22 November 2002). Available under the Timeline entry for November 22, 2002, at http://www.miami.edu/ethics/schiavo/schiavo_timeline.html.
22. Kenney, R., and Dellert, C. Commentary 2: The Schiavo case was exploited for dramatic effect. *Journal of Mass Media Ethics* 2006;21(2&3):219–222.
23. Caplan, A. Commentary 3: The Schiavo case was one of the greatest failures of the American media. *Journal of Mass Media Ethics* 21(2&3):223–228.
24. Ibid.
25. Boehlert, E. A tale told by an idiot. www.Salon.com, March 31, 2005. Available at: http://dir.salon.com/story/news/feature/2005/03/31/schiavo_media/index.html.

26. Squires, T. On Schiavo case, TV struggles for balance. *St. Petersburg Times/ONLINE/TAMPA BAY,* April 1, 2005. Available at: http://www.sptimes.com/2005/04/01/news_pf/Tampabay/ On_Schiavo_case__TV_s.shtml.

27. Douglas, "Commentary 1: Duke Righteous meets Terri Schiavo."

28. *Schindler v Schiavo,* 851 So 2d 182, 187 (Fla. Dist. Ct. App. 2003) at p. 10. Available under the Timeline entry for June 6, 2003, at: http://www.miami.edu/ethics/schiavo/schiavo_timeline.html.

29. Murrow, E.R. Address to the Radio Television News Directors Association, October 15, 1958. Transcript available at: http://www.turnoffyourtv.com/commentary/hiddenagenda/murrow.html.

APPENDIX ⠶

Timeline of Key Events in the Case of Theresa Marie Schiavo

This resource is maintained at http://www.miami.edu/ethics/schiavo/schiavo_timeline.html. Please refer to this website for credits and acknowledgments. The on-line resource includes links to key legal documents and selected news reports.

DECEMBER 3, 1963

Theresa (Terri) Marie Schindler is born in Pennsylvania.

NOVEMBER 10, 1984

Terri Schindler, 20, and Michael Schiavo, 21, are married at Our Lady of Good Counsel Church in Southampton, Pennsylvania. The union is now among the "celebrity marriages" featured at About.com, a website about marriage.

1986

The couple move to St. Petersburg, where Ms. Schiavo's parents had retired.

FEBRUARY 25, 1990

Ms. Schiavo suffers cardiac arrest, apparently caused by a potassium imbalance and leading to brain damage due to lack of oxygen. She was taken to the Humana Northside Hospital and was later given a percutaneous endoscopic gastrostomy (PEG) to provide nutrition and hydration.

MAY 12, 1990

Ms. Schiavo is discharged from the hospital and taken to the College Park skilled care and rehabilitation facility.

JUNE 18, 1990

Court appoints Michael Schiavo as guardian; Ms. Schiavo's parents do not object.

JUNE 30, 1990

Ms. Schiavo is transferred to Bayfront Hospital for further rehabilitation efforts.

SEPTEMBER 1990

Ms. Schiavo's family brings her home, but three weeks later they return her to the College Park facility because the family is "overwhelmed by Terri's care needs."

NOVEMBER 1990

Michael Schiavo takes Ms. Schiavo to California for experimental "brain stimulator" treatment, an experimental "thalamic stimulator implant" in her brain.

JANUARY 1991

The Schiavos return to Florida; Ms. Schiavo is moved to the Mediplex Rehabilitation Center in Brandon, where she receives 24-hour care.

JULY 19, 1991

Ms. Schiavo is transferred to Sable Palms skilled care facility, where she receives continuing neurological testing and regular and aggressive speech/occupational therapy through 1994.

MAY 1992

Ms. Schiavo's parents, Robert and Mary Schindler, and Michael Schiavo stop living together.

AUGUST 1992

Ms. Schiavo is awarded $250,000 in an out-of-court medical malpractice settlement with one of her physicians.

NOVEMBER 1992

The jury in the medical malpractice trial against another of Ms. Schiavo's physicians awards more than $1 million dollars. In the end, after attorneys' fees and other expenses, Michael Schiavo received about $300,000 and about $750,000 was put in a trust fund specifically for Ms. Schiavo's medical care.

FEBRUARY 14, 1993

Michael Schiavo and the Schindlers have a falling-out over the course of therapy for Ms. Schiavo; Michael Schiavo claims that the Schindlers demand that he share the malpractice money with them.

JULY 29, 1993

The Schindlers attempt to remove Michael Schiavo as Ms. Schiavo's guardian; the court later dismisses the suit.

MARCH 1, 1994

First guardian ad litem, John H. Pecarek, submits his report. He states that Michael Schiavo has acted appropriately and attentively toward Ms. Schiavo.

MAY 6, 1997

Michael Schiavo's attorney Deborah Bushnell writes to the Circuit Court to request that the Schindlers receive notice of all filings in the guardianship proceeding, in anticipation of a forthcoming request to withdraw Ms. Schiavo's PEG tube.

MAY 1998

Michael Schiavo petitions the court to authorize the removal of Ms. Schiavo's PEG tube; the Schindlers oppose, saying that she would want to remain alive. The court appoints Richard Pearse, Esq., to serve as the second guardian ad litem for Ms. Schiavo.

DECEMBER 20, 1998

The second guardian ad litem, Richard Pearse, Esq., issues his report, in which he concludes that Ms. Schiavo is in a persistent vegetative state with no chance of improvement and that Michael Schiavo's decision making may be influenced by the potential to inherit the remainder of Ms. Schiavo's estate.

JANUARY 24, 2000

The trial begins; Pinellas-Pasco County Circuit Court Judge George Greer presides.

FEBRUARY 11, 2000

Judge Greer rules that Ms. Schiavo would have chosen to have the PEG tube removed, and therefore he orders it removed, which, according to doctors, will cause her death in approximately 7 to 14 days.

MARCH 2, 2000

The Schindlers file a petition with Judge Greer to allow "swallowing" tests to be performed on Ms. Schiavo to determine if she can consume—or learn to consume—nutrients on her own.

MARCH 7, 2000

Judge Greer denies the Schindlers' petition to perform "swallowing" tests on Ms. Schiavo.

MARCH 24, 2000

Judge Greer grants Michael Schiavo's petition to limit visitation to Ms. Schiavo as well as to bar pictures. Judge Greer also stays his order until 30 days beyond the final exhaustion of all appeals by the Schindlers.

JANUARY 24, 2001

Florida's Second District Court of Appeal (2nd DCA) upholds Judge Greer's ruling that permits the removal of Ms. Schiavo's PEG tube.

In re Schiavo, 780 So. 2d 176 (2nd DCA 2001), *rehearing denied* (Feb. 22, 2001), *review denied*, 789 So. 2d 348 (Fla. 2001). (Case No.: SC01-559)

FEBRUARY 22, 2001

The Schindler family's motion for an Appellate Court rehearing is denied.

MARCH 12, 2001

Michael Schiavo petitions Judge Greer to lift his stay, issued March 24, 2000, in order to permit the removal of Ms. Schiavo's PEG tube.

MARCH 29, 2001

Judge Greer denies Michael Schiavo's motion to lift stay issued on March 24, 2000; Michael Schiavo can remove Ms. Schiavo's PEG tube at 1 p.m. on April 20.

APRIL 10, 2001

The 2nd DCA denies the Schindlers' motion to extend Judge Greer's stay, which is scheduled to expire April 20, 2001.

APRIL 12, 2001

The Schindlers file a motion requesting that Judge Greer recuse himself.
The Schindlers petition the Florida Supreme Court to stay the removal of Ms. Schiavo's PEG tube.

APRIL 16, 2001

Judge Greer denies the Schindlers' motion to recuse himself.

APRIL 18, 2001

The Florida Supreme Court chooses not to review the decision of the 2nd DCA. *In re* Schiavo, 789 So. 2d 248 (Fla. 2001). Case No.: SC01-559

APRIL 20, 2001

Federal District Court Judge Richard Lazzara grants the Schindlers a stay until April 23, 2001, to exhaust all their possible appeals.

APRIL 23, 2001

Justice Anthony M. Kennedy of the United States Supreme Court refuses to stay the case for a review by that Court.

APRIL 24, 2001

By order of trial court Judge Greer, and upon issuance of a 2nd DCA mandate, Ms. Schiavo's PEG tube is removed.

APRIL 26, 2001

The Schindlers file an emergency motion with Judge Greer for relief from judgment based upon new evidence, which includes a claim that a former girlfriend of Michael Schiavo will testify that he lied about Ms. Schiavo's wishes; Judge Greer dismisses the motion as untimely. Also on this date, the Schindlers file a new civil suit that claims that Michael Schiavo perjured himself when he testified that Ms. Schiavo had stated an aversion to remaining on life support. Pending this new civil trial, Circuit Court Judge Frank Quesada orders Ms. Schiavo's PEG tube to be reinserted.

APRIL 30, 2001

Michael Schiavo files an emergency motion with the 2nd DCA to allow the removal of Ms. Schiavo's PEG tube.

MAY 9, 2001

The 2nd DCA announces a date for the hearing of oral arguments regarding Michael Schiavo's motion of April 30, 2001.

JUNE 25, 2001

Arguments in 2nd DCA regarding Michael Schiavo's motion of April 30, 2001.

JULY 11, 2001

The 2nd DCA remands the case back to Judge Greer. (1) The 2nd DCA informs the Schindlers that they must address both their desire to have new evidence heard and their perjury claim against Michael Schiavo within the original guardianship proceeding; further, the Schindlers are instructed to file a new motion for relief from judgment in the guardianship proceeding. (2) The 2nd DCA instructs Judge Greer to weigh the Schindlers' new evidence in making a new determination of what Ms. Schiavo would have wanted. (3) The 2nd DCA denies Michael Schiavo's request to discontinue the PEG tube. *In re Schiavo*, 792 So. 2d 551 (2nd DCA 2001).

AUGUST 7, 2001

After the 2nd DCA remands the case back to Judge Greer, he again finds that Michael Schiavo may remove Ms. Schiavo's PEG tube on August 28.

AUGUST 10, 2001

Judge Greer denies the Schindlers' motion (1) to have their own doctors examine Ms. Schiavo, (2) to remove Michael Schiavo as her guardian, and (3) to disqualify himself from the proceedings.

AUGUST 17, 2001

Judge Greer delays the removal of Ms. Schiavo's PEG tube until October 9 in order to allow the Schindlers time to appeal.

OCTOBER 3, 2001

The 2nd DCA delays the removal of the PEG tube indefinitely.

OCTOBER 17, 2001

The 2nd DCA rules that five doctors should examine Ms. Schiavo to determine if she can improve with new medical treatment. The Schindlers and Michael Schiavo are to choose two doctors each, and the court is to appoint a doctor. The appeals court also affirms Greer's denial of the motion to disqualify himself. *In re Schiavo*, 800 So. 2d 640 (2nd DCA 2001).

NOVEMBER 1, 2001

The 2nd DCA denies Michael Schiavo's motion to rehear the case.

DECEMBER 14, 2001

Michael Schiavo petitions the Florida Supreme Court to stay the October 17, 2001, ruling of the 2nd DCA. He states that he and the Schindlers will attempt to mediate the dispute in lieu of further litigation.

DECEMBER 19, 2001

Attorneys meet with a mediator to determine which tests doctors should run on Ms. Schiavo.

JANUARY 10, 2002

State Supreme Court stays all legal proceedings pending mediation; it orders attorneys to report on the status of mediation in 60 days.

FEBRUARY 13, 2002

Mediation between the Schindlers and Michael Schiavo fails.

MARCH 14, 2002

The Florida Supreme Court denies Michael Schiavo's petition to review the 2nd DCA's ruling allowing five doctors to examine Ms. Schiavo. *In re Schiavo*, 816 So. 2d 127 (Fla. 2002) (Table, No. SC01-2678)

OCTOBER 12-22, 2002

The trial court holds a new hearing on new potential medical treatments.

NOVEMBER 15, 2002

The Schindlers contend that Michael Schiavo might have abused Ms. Schiavo and this abuse led to her condition. They ask the court for more time to collect evidence, and to remove Michael Schiavo as guardian.

NOVEMBER 22, 2002

Judge Greer rules that Ms. Schiavo's PEG tube should be removed January 3, 2003. *In re Schiavo*, 2002 WL 31817960 (Fla. Cir. Ct. Nov. 22, 2002) (No. 90-2908-GB-003)

DECEMBER 13, 2002

Judge Greer stays his November 22 ruling: Ms. Schiavo should not have her PEG tube removed until an appeals court can rule on the case.

DECEMBER 23, 2002

The 2nd DCA denies a motion Michael Schiavo filed seeking permission to remove the PEG tube.

JUNE 6, 2003

The 2nd DCA, affirming Judge Greer's November 2002 ruling, concludes that Michael Schiavo can remove Ms. Schiavo's PEG tube on October 15. *In re Schiavo*, 851 So. 2d 182 (2nd DCA 2003) (No. 2D02-5394), *rehearing denied* (July 9, 2003), *review denied* 855 So. 2d 621 (Fla. 2003).

JULY 9, 2003

The 2nd DCA refuses to reconsider its decision.

AUGUST 22, 2003

The Florida Supreme Court declines to review the decision. *Schindler v. Schiavo*, 855 So. 2d 621 (Fla. 2003) (Table, No. SC03-1242)

AUGUST 30, 2003

Ms. Schiavo's parents file a federal lawsuit challenging the removal of Ms. Schiavo's PEG tube. Schiavos' petition (D). *Schindler v. Schiavo, Civil Action No. 8:03-CV-1860-T-26-T-TGW*

SEPTEMBER 17, 2003

Judge Greer orders the removal of the PEG tube to take place on October 15, 2003. He also rejects the Schindlers' request that Ms. Schiavo be given therapy to learn how to eat without the tube.

OCTOBER 7, 2003

Governor Jeb Bush files a federal court brief in support of the Schindlers' effort to stop the removal of the PEG tube.

OCTOBER 10, 2003

Federal Court Judge Richard Lazzara rules that he lacks the jurisdiction to hear the federal case.

OCTOBER 14, 2003

The 2nd DCA refuses to block Judge Greer's order to remove the PEG tube.

OCTOBER 15, 2003

Ms. Schiavo's PEG tube is once again removed.

OCTOBER 17, 2003

The Florida Circuit Court in Pinellas County and the First District Court of Appeal refuse to grant a request by "supporters" of the Schindlers to direct Gov. Bush to intervene in the case.

OCTOBER 19, 2003

The Advocacy Center for Persons with Disabilities, Inc. files a federal court lawsuit that claims that the removal of Ms. Schiavo's PEG tube is abuse and neglect.

Advocacy Center for Persons with Disabilities, Inc. v. Schiavo, No. 8:03-CV-2167-T-23EAJ

OCTOBER 20, 2003

The Florida House of Representatives passes a bill, "Terri's Law," that allows the governor to issue a "one-time stay in certain cases."

OCTOBER 21, 2003

The Florida Senate passes the bill; Governor Bush issues an executive order directing reinsertion of the PEG tube and appointing a guardian ad litem for Ms. Schiavo.

Michael Schiavo files a state-court lawsuit arguing that "Terri's Law" is unconstitutional and seeking an injunction to stop the reinsertion of the PEG tube; the court requests briefs on the Constitutional arguments about "Terri's Law." *Schiavo v. Bush.* No. 03-008212-CI-20 (Cir. Ct. Pinellas County, Florida).

The federal court denies the motion for a temporary restraining order filed in the lawsuit of the Advocacy Center for Persons with Disabilities, Inc. *Advocacy Center for Persons with Disabilities, Inc. v. Schiavo*, 2003 WL 23305833, 17 Fla. L. Weekly Fed. D 291 (M.D. Fla. Oct. 21, 2003).

Ms. Schiavo's PEG tube is reinserted.

OCTOBER 22, 2003

David Demers, Chief Judge for the Pinellas County Circuit Court, orders both the Schindlers and Michael Schiavo to agree within 5 days on an independent guardian ad litem as required under the Governor's order. ("Terri's Law" directs: "Upon issuance of the stay, the chief judge of the circuit court shall appoint a guardian ad litem for the patient to make recommendations to the Governor and the court.")

OCTOBER 28, 2003

President George W. Bush praises the way his brother, Governor Jeb Bush, has handled the Schiavo matter.

OCTOBER 29, 2003

Michael Schiavo files court papers in his state-court lawsuit, arguing that "Terri's Law" is unconstitutional. The American Civil Liberties Union has joined Michael Schiavo.

OCTOBER 31, 2003

Judge Demers appoints Prof. Jay Wolfson as Ms. Schiavo's guardian ad litem. Dr. Wolfson holds both medical and legal degrees; he is also a public health professor at the University of South Florida. He is supposed to represent Ms. Schiavo's best interests in court, but he has no authority to make decisions for her.

NOVEMBER 4, 2003

Governor Jeb Bush asks Circuit Court Judge W. Douglas Baird to dismiss Michael Schiavo's suit (filed October 21, 2003) that challenges "Terri's Law."

NOVEMBER 8, 2003

Judge Baird denies Governor Bush's motion to dismiss the state-court suit.

NOVEMBER 10, 2003

Governor Bush appeals Judge Baird's decision; the filing of the appeal has the effect of staying the removal of Ms. Schiavo's PEG tube.

NOVEMBER 14, 2003

Judge Baird vacates the stay.

NOVEMBER 14, 2003

In response to Judge Baird's lifting the stay, the 2nd DCA issues an indefinite stay.

NOVEMBER 19, 2003

Governor Bush files a petition to remove Judge Baird.

NOVEMBER 21, 2003

Florida Sens. Stephen Wise and Jim Sebesta introduce legislation (S692) that would require persons in persistent vegetative states to be administered medically supplied nutrition and hydration in the absence of a living will, regardless of family beliefs about what those patients would have wanted. The measure is withdrawn from consideration on April 16, 2004.

DECEMBER 1, 2003

University of South Florida Prof. Jay Wolfson, guardian ad litem, concludes in his report that Ms. Schiavo is in a persistent vegetative state with no chance of improvement.

DECEMBER 10, 2003

The 2nd DCA refuses to remove Judge Baird, who is the presiding judge in the state-court lawsuit filed October 21, 2003. *Bush v. Schiavo*, 861 So. 2d 506 (2nd DCA 2003) (No. 2D03-5244)

JANUARY 5, 2004

The Schindler family petitions the Pinellas County Circuit Court to reappoint Prof. Wolfson the guardian ad litem.

JANUARY 8, 2004

Judge Demers rejects the request to reappoint the guardian ad litem, citing the pending court decisions over the constitutionality of "Terri's Law" as reason to wait on any action.

FEBRUARY 13, 2004

The 2nd DCA reverses Judge Baird's ruling (in the case filed October 21, 2003) that denied the Schindlers permission to intervene in Michael Schiavo's Constitutional challenge to "Terri's Law." The 2nd DCA explains that Judge Baird did not follow proper procedure. The court also gives permission to Governor Bush to question several witnesses who Judge Baird previously had ruled could not offer any relevant testimony. *Bush v. Schiavo*, 866 So. 2d 140 (Fla. 2nd DCA 2004) (on intervention); 866 So. 2d 136 (2nd DCA 2004) (on request to take depositions). (Case No. 2D03-5783).

MARCH 12, 2004

Judge Baird again rejects the Schindlers' request to intervene in Michael Schiavo's suit that questions the constitutionality of "Terri's Law."

MARCH 20, 2004

Pope John Paul II addresses World Federation of Catholic Medical Associations and Pontifical Academy for Life Congress on "Life-Sustaining Treatments and Vegetative State: Scientific Advances and Ethical Dilemmas." His remarks spark widespread interest and controversy.

MARCH 29, 2004

Nursing home workers discover four "fresh puncture wounds" on one arm and a fifth wound on the other arm; the workers state that a hypodermic needle appears to have caused the wounds. Attendants discovered the wounds shortly after the Schindlers visited Ms. Schiavo for 45 minutes. Toxicology reports indicate that no substance was injected into Ms. Schiavo. Clearwater police later conclude that the marks might have been made by a device used to move Ms. Schiavo and, in any case, that no evidence of abuse or other wrongdoing could be found.

MARCH 29, 2004

Judge Greer denies a motion filed by the Schindlers seeking to have Michael Schiavo defend himself in a hearing; they allege that he is violating a 1996 court order that requires him to share a sufficient amount of Ms. Schiavo's medical information. Michael Schiavo claims that he has shared an adequate amount of information through attorneys.

APRIL 16, 2004

S692 is withdrawn from consideration in the Florida Legislature.

APRIL 23, 2004

The 2nd DCA rules that the Pinellas County trial court has jurisdiction to hear and is the proper venue for the case Michael Schiavo has filed against Governor Bush asserting that "Terri's Law" is unconstitutional.

MAY 5, 2004

Pinellas Circuit Judge W. Douglas Baird rules that "Terri's Law," sought and signed by Gov. Bush and approved by the Legislature on October 21, 2003, is unconstitutional. The governor appeals the ruling.

JUNE 1, 2004

The 2nd DCA grants a motion from attorneys for Michael Schiavo to send the case directly to the Florida Supreme Court and bypass a lower-court review. Meanwhile, attorneys for Gov. Bush file a motion asking that all appeals be halted until the issue of whether Michael Schiavo has the authority to fight the governor on his wife's behalf is resolved.

JUNE 16, 2004

Florida's Supreme Court, pointing to "a question of great public importance requiring immediate resolution by this Court," accepts jurisdiction and sets oral arguments for August 31, 2004.

JUNE 30, 2004

2nd DCA affirms Judge Baird's March 12 ruling denying the Schindlers the ability to intervene in the lawsuit over the constitutionality of "Terri's Law."

JULY 19, 2004

The Schindlers file a motion in the Circuit Court for Pinellas County seeking relief from judgment in *Schindler v. Schiavo*. Based in part upon the recent statement by Pope John Paul II, they argue that the orders mandating withdrawal of the PEG tube from Ms. Schiavo and authorizing Michael to challenge the constitutionality of "Terri's Law" violate her "free exercise of her religious beliefs [and] her right to enjoy and defend her own life and, in fact, imperil her immortal soul."

JULY 27, 2004

National group of bioethicists files *amicus* brief "in support of Michael Schiavo as guardian of the person."

AUGUST 31, 2004

The Florida Supreme Court hears oral arguments in the lawsuit over the constitutionality of "Terri's Law."

AUGUST 31, 2004

Circuit Judge George Greer, opposed for re-election by an attorney who was known to oppose Greer's rulings in the Schiavo case, is re-elected by a large margin.

SEPTEMBER 23, 2004

Florida's Supreme Court, unanimously affirming the trial court order, declares "Terri's Law" unconstitutional.

OCTOBER 4, 2004

Governor Bush files a motion and then an amended motion for rehearing and clarification of the Florida Supreme Court opinion issued on September 23, 2004

OCTOBER 21, 2004

Florida Supreme Court denies Governor Bush's amended motion for rehearing and clarification, as well as a motion seeking permission to file a second amended motion for rehearing and clarification. The Court issues a mandate to transfer jurisdiction back to Judge Greer.

OCTOBER 22, 2004

In Pinellas County, at the trial-court level, Judge Greer denies the motion filed by the Schindlers on July 19, 2004. He also stays the removal of her PEG tube until December 6, 2004.

OCTOBER 25, 2004

Governor Bush files a motion with the Florida Supreme Court asking that it recall the mandate it issued on October 22 because he will be filing a petition for *certiorari* regarding this case with the U.S. Supreme Court.

OCTOBER 27, 2004

Florida Supreme Court grants Governor Bush's motion asking that it recall the mandate issued on October 22. Proceedings in the trial and all appellate courts in the case of *Bush v. Schiavo* are stayed until November 29, 2004.

NOVEMBER 22, 2004

In the guardianship proceeding in Pinellas County, the Schindlers appeal from Judge Greer's October 22 order denying their motion for relief from judgment.

DECEMBER 1, 2004

Governor Bush files a petition for *certiorari*, seeking review of the Florida Supreme Court's decision regarding "Terri's Law," with the U.S. Supreme Court.

DECEMBER 29, 2004

2nd DCA, without opinion, denies the Schindlers' November 22 appeal from Judge Greer's order refusing to reopen the guardianship proceeding.

JANUARY 10, 2005

The Schindlers again ask Judge Greer to remove Michael Schiavo from his judicial appointed post of Ms. Schiavo's guardian.

JANUARY 13, 2005

The Schindlers file two motions—one in the 2nd DCA, asking it to reconsider its decision of December 29, 2004, and a second in the trial court guardianship proceeding, asking Judge Greer once again to prevent withdrawal of nutrition and hydration until the 2nd DCA does so.

JANUARY 24, 2005

The U.S. Supreme Court refuses to grant review of the case in which the Florida Supreme Court struck down "Terri's Law" as unconstitutional.

FEBRUARY 7, 2005

Florida's Department of Agriculture and Consumer Services cites the Terri Schindler-Schiavo Foundation for failing to register with the state to solicit donations.

FEBRUARY 11, 2005

In Pinellas County, Judge Greer denies the Schindlers' motions, filed January 10 and 13, 2005. The order authorizing withdrawal of the PEG tube remains in effect, although implementation is stayed pending the outcome of currently pending appeals.

FEBRUARY 15, 2005

The Schindlers ask the 2nd DCA to stay the mandate issued when it refused to hear their most recent appeal.

FEBRUARY 16, 2005

Randall Terry, founder of the pro-life activist organization Operation Rescue, appears with the Schindlers at a news conference, vowing protest vigils against removal of the PEG tube.

FEBRUARY 18, 2005

The Schindlers again petition Judge Greer in Pinellas County for reconsideration of the order of February 11, 2005, in which the court upheld its judgment, made in the year 2000, that the PEG tube should be removed.

FEBRUARY 18, 2005

Florida Representatives Baxley Brown; Cannon; Davis, D.; Flores; Goldstein; Lopez-Cantera; Murzin; Quinones; Traviesa introduce H.701 in the Florida Legislature. H.701, mirroring S.692 (introduced in October 2003 and withdrawn in April 2004), would require maintenance of medically supplied nutrition and hydration in incapacitated persons in most instances.

FEBRUARY 21, 2005

The 2d DCA denies the Schindlers' motion of February 15, 2005, clearing the way for removal of the PEG tube when the current stay expires on February 22, 2005. Judge Greer schedules a hearing on the Schindlers' motion of February 18, 2005, for February 23, 2005.

FEBRUARY 22, 2005

Judge Greer stays removal of the PEG tube until 5 p.m. on February 23, 2005 (after he hears argument on the motion filed by the Schindlers on February 18, 2005).

FEBRUARY 23, 2005

After a hearing, Judge Greer extends the stay preventing removal of the PEG tube until 5 p.m. on February 25, 2005, to permit time to issue an order detailing his decisions regarding matters discussed at the hearing. Officials from Florida's Department of Children and Families (DCF) move to intervene in the case, but Judge Greer denies the motion to intervene at the hearing.

FEBRUARY 25, 2005

Judge Greer denies the motion before him and orders that, "absent a stay from the appellate courts, the guardian, Michael Schiavo, shall cause the removal of nutrition and hydration from the ward, Theresa Schiavo, at 1 p.m. on Friday, March 18, 2005."

FEBRUARY 26, 2005

The *St. Petersburg Times* reports that a Vatican cardinal spoke on Vatican Radio opposing removal of the PEG tube.

FEBRUARY 28, 2005

The Schindlers file a number of motions with Judge Greer, addressing a range of issues. They also indicate that they will appeal the judge's decision of February 25, 2005. Judge Greer denies some of the motions but agrees to set a hearing date to consider others.

MARCH 7, 2005

The Schindlers appeal Judge Greer's February 25, 2005, order to the 2nd DCA. Bioethicists from six Florida universities submit an analysis of H.701.

MARCH 8, 2005

U.S. Rep. David Weldon (R-Fla.) introduces in the United States House of Representatives H.R. 1151, titled the Incapacitated Persons' Legal Protection Act. The bill would permit a federal court to review the Schiavo matter through a *habeas corpus* lawsuit.

MARCH 9, 2005

The Florida House Health Care Regulation Committee considers H.701, voting to approve a Council/Committee Substitute 701 instead of the original version.

MARCH 10, 2005

Judge Greer issues order denying Florida's Department of Children and Families the right to intervene in the guardianship case.

MARCH 14, 2005

The Judiciary Committee in the Florida House considers H.701, voting to approve another Committee substitute for the original bill. The *South Florida Sun-Sentinel* reports that the House and the Senate have agreed that this bill will come to a vote.

The Florida House Health & Families Council considers and approves the second committee substitute H.701.

The Florida Senate Judiciary Committee passes S.804, providing that medically supplied nutrition and hydration cannot be "suspended from" a person in a PVS if: (1) the purpose of the suspension is "solely to end the life of" a person in a PVS; (2) a conflict exists on the issue of suspension of medically supplied nutrition and hydration among the persons who could be proxy decisionmakers for that person under Florida law; and (3) the person in the PVS had not executed a written advance directive or designated a health care surrogate.

The 2nd DCA affirms Judge Greer's orders and refuses to stay the scheduled March 18 withdrawal of the PEG tube.

The U.S. House of Representatives, by voice vote, passes H.R. 1332, the Protection of Incapacitated Persons Act of 2005. This bill would amend federal law to provide for removal of certain cases to federal court from state court, rather than authorizing use of the federal *habeas corpus* remedy to obtain federal court review, as H.R. 1151 would have.

The Florida House of Representatives approves H.701, after some amendments.

The Florida Senate votes down S.804.

Florida's Department of Children and Families (DCF) petitions the Florida Supreme Court for relief, and the Florida Supreme Court denies the petition.The U.S. Senate passes a "private bill" applying to the Schiavo case but differing from H.R. 1332. The U.S. Senate website, at www.senate.gov, explains a "private bill" as follows: "A private bill provides benefits to specified individuals (including corporate bodies). Individuals sometimes request relief through private legislation when administrative or legal remedies are exhausted. Many private bills deal with immigration—granting citizenship or permanent residency. Private bills may also be introduced for individuals who have claims again the government, veterans' benefits claims, claims for military decorations, or taxation problems. The title of a private bill usually begins with the phrase, "For the relief of. . . ." If a private bill is passed in identical form by both houses of Congress and is signed by the President, it becomes a private law."

The Schindlers ask the U.S. Supreme Court to hear the case, but the U.S. Supreme Court denies their petition.

Republican senators circulate a memo on the political advantages of supporting legislation to reinsert Ms. Schiavo's nutrition tube. On April 7, *The Washington Post* reported that "The legal counsel to Sen. Mel Martinez (R-Fla.) admitted [on April 6] that he was the author of a memo citing the political advantage to Republicans of intervening in the case . . . Brian H. Darling, 39, a former lobbyist for the Alexander Strategy Group on gun rights and other issues, offered his resignation and it was immediately accepted, Martinez said."

MARCH 18, 2005

The U.S. House of Representatives Committee on Government Reform issues five subpoenas: one commanding Michael Schiavo to appear before it and bring with him the "hydration and nutrition equipment" in working order; three commanding physicians and other personnel at the hospice to do the same; and one commanding Ms. Schiavo to appear before it. The subpoenas would require that the PEG tube remain in working order until at least the date of testimony, March 25, 2005. The subpoenas are included as appendices to the U.S. House All Writs Petition (see just below).

The Committee on Government Reform also moves to intervene in the guardianship litigation before Judge Greer and asks Judge Greer to stay his order requiring removal of the PEG tube. Judge Greer denies the motions.

The Committee on Government Reform files an emergency all-writs petition with the Florida Supreme Court, effectively seeking reversal of Judge Greer's denial of its motions. The Florida Supreme Court denies this petition.

The House Committee on Government Reform asks the U.S. Supreme Court to review the Florida Supreme Court's denial of its petition. Justice Kennedy, acting for the Court, denies the application for relief.

The PEG tube is removed in mid-afternoon. This is the third time the tube has been removed in accordance with court orders.

The Schindlers, as "next friends" of their daughter, file a petition for writ of *habeas corpus* in federal district court in the Middle District of Florida. That court dismisses the case for lack of jurisdiction and refuses to issue a temporary restraining order because "there is not a substantial likelihood that [the Schindlers] will prevail on their federal constitutional claims."

MARCH 19-20, 2005

The U.S. Senate delays its Easter recess and works on Saturday to reach a compromise with the House on a bill, S.686, closely resembling the special bill it passed on March 17. On Palm Sunday (which holiday is frequently noted in debate), it then passes S.686 and the U.S. House of Representatives returns from Easter recess for a special session to debate S.686.

MARCH 20, 2005

House Democrats and Republicans hold news conferences.

MARCH 21, 2005

Shortly past 12:30 a.m., the U.S. House of Representatives votes 203–58 to suspend its rules and pass S.686.

President Bush signs S.686 at 1:11 a.m.

Federal District Court Judge James D. Whittemore, Middle District of Florida (in Tampa), hears arguments on the Schindlers' motion that he order re-insertion of the PEG tube while the lawsuit they will assert pursuant to S.686 is litigated.

MARCH 22, 2005

Federal District Court Judge Whittemore refuses to order re-insertion of the PEG tube.

The Schindlers appeal Judge Whittemore's decision to the U.S. Court of Appeals for the Eleventh Circuit.

The Schindlers file an amended complaint in the federal district court, adding a number of new claims.

MARCH 23, 2005

The U.S. Eleventh Circuit Court of Appeals, in a 2–1 vote, denies the Schindlers' appeal.United States Eleventh Circuit Court of Appeals, acting *en banc* (as a whole), refuses to rehear the Schindlers' appeal, leaving intact the court's ruling earlier in the day.

House Democrats and Republicans hold news conferences.

The Florida Senate, by a vote of 21–18, again refuses to pass S.804. This bill was approved by the Senate Judiciary Committee on March 15, 2005.

Florida Governor Jeb Bush reports that a neurologist, Dr. William Cheshire, claims that Ms. Schiavo is not in a persistent vegetative state. The governor asks the Florida Department of Children and Families (DCF) to obtain custody of Ms. Schiavo in light of allegations of abuse. Judge Greer holds a hearing on the matter.

The Schindlers file a petition for writ of *certiorari* with the U.S. Supreme Court.

Judge Greer issues a restraining order prohibiting DCF from removing Ms. Schiavo from the hospice or otherwise re-inserting the PEG tube.

The Schindlers ask again for a restraining order in federal court.

Five members of the U.S. House of Representatives ask the U.S. Supreme Court to file a "friend of the court" brief.

MARCH 24, 2005

The U.S. Supreme Court refuses to hear the Schindlers' case. The Schindlers file a Second Amended Complaint, adding several claims, in the federal court case. Count X, titled "Right to Life," alleges a violation of the Fourteenth Amendment's right to life because removing the PEG tube is "contrary to [Ms. Schiavo's] wish to live."

The trial court (Judge Whittemore) schedules a hearing for 6 p.m. and orders supplemental briefs on Count X.

Judge Greer denies DCF's motion to intervene. DCF appeals Judge Greer's order. Judge Greer vacates the automatic stay upon appeal. The 2nd District Court of Appeal refuses to reinstate the stay. The Florida Supreme Court dismisses a motion on this matter because it "fails to invoke" the court's jurisdiction.

MARCH 25, 2005

Judge Whittemore denies the Schindlers' second motion for an order re-inserting the PEG tube.

The Schindlers appeal Judge Whittemore's order to the U.S. Court of Appeals for the Eleventh Circuit. The Eleventh Circuit affirms. The Schindlers announce that they will pursue no more federal appeals.

The Schindlers file an emergency motion attempting to convince Judge Greer to reinsert the PEG, at least temporarily until the Eleventh Circuit decides their appeal. The motion contends her family heard her try to verbalize "I want to live," according to news reports. (This motion and accompanying affidavits make up Appendix 7 of the Schindlers' Petition linked under March 26, just below.)

DCF appeals Judge Greer's March 23 denial of its first motion to intervene to the 2nd DCA.

MARCH 26, 2005

Judge Greer denies the Schindlers' motion of March 25, 2005.
The Schindlers appeal to the Florida Supreme Court to reverse Judge Greer's refusal to reinsert the PEG tube, but the Florida Supreme Court refuses to do so, citing a lack of jurisdiction.

News agencies report the arrest on March 25 of Richard Alan Meywes of Fairview, N.C., for offering $250,000 for the killing of Michael Schiavo and another $50,000 for the death of Judge Greer. After serving 31 days in jail he was sentenced to 18 months probation, from which he was released after 13 months.

The Schindlers advise supporters demonstrating around the hospice to return home to spend the Easter holiday with their families. The protesters remain.

MARCH 27, 2005

In an interview on CNN, Governor Bush says: "I cannot violate a court order. I don't have power from the U.S. Constitution, or the Florida Constitution for that matter, that would allow me to intervene after a decision has been made."

MARCH 29, 2005

The Rev. Jesse Jackson leads a prayer service outside the hospice and speaks out against removal of the PEG tube.

The 2nd DCA upholds Judge Greer's ruling refusing to let the DCF intervene.

Despite earlier indications that they would pursue no further federal appeals, the Schindlers petition the entire Eleventh Circuit Court of Appeals for permission to file a motion for rehearing *en banc* although the time to do so has expired. A grant of that petition would enable the Schindlers to ask for review of the Eleventh Circuit decision of March 24.

March 30, 2005

The Eleventh Circuit permits the Schindlers' filing and then, acting both through a panel and as a whole, denies the motion for rehearing.

The U.S. Supreme Court refuses to review the Eleventh Circuit ruling.

MARCH 31, 2005

Ms. Schiavo dies at 9:05 a.m. Her body is transported to the Pinellas Country Coroner's Office for an autopsy.

Judge Greer authorizes Michael Schiavo to administer Ms. Schiavo's estate.

On this date in 1976, the New Jersey Supreme Court ruled that coma patient Karen Ann Quinlan could be disconnected from her respirator. She remained in a persistent vegetative state and died in 1985.

APRIL 12, 2005

The Wall Street Journal Online/Harris Interactive Health Care Poll finds that "most people disapprove of how President Bush, Governor Bush, and the Congress handled the issue."

APRIL 15, 2005

In response to a motion from the media, Judge Greer orders DCF to release redacted copies of abuse reports regarding Ms. Schiavo. Newspapers report that DCF found no evidence of abuse after investigating the 89 reports filed before February 18, 2005. Thirty allegations are outstanding and still being investigated, but Judge Greer earlier had ruled that those allegations duplicated those previously filed.

MAY 17, 2005

More than six weeks after Ms. Schiavo's death, Lisa Wilson is the last of the hundreds of protesters outside Ms. Schiavo's hospice.

JUNE 15, 2005

Dr. Jon Thogmartin, Florida's District Six Medical Examiner, releases the results of Ms. Schiavo's autopsy. He reports that the autopsy showed Ms. Schiavo's condition was "consistent" with a person in a persistent vegetative state. "This damage was irreversible," he said. "No amount of therapy or treatment would have regenerated the massive loss of neurons." No evidence of abuse was found, he said.

JUNE 17, 2005

Florida Governor Jeb Bush asks a state prosecutor to investigate the circumstances of Ms. Schiavo's 1990 cardiac arrest, specifically the amount of time that elapsed between the time Ms. Schiavo collapsed and Michael Schiavo called 911.

JUNE 20, 2005

Despite earlier statements that he intended to bury Ms. Schiavo's remains in Pennsylvania, Michael Schiavo buries them in Clearwater, Florida. The grave marker reads:

Schiavo
Theresa Marie

Beloved Wife
Born December 3, 1963
Departed This Earth
February 25, 1990
At Peace MARCH 31, 2005

I Kept My Promise

JUNE 22, 2005

News organizations report that Randall Terry, leader of a pro-life group that demonstrated against removal of Ms. Schiavo's PEG tube, intends to run for Florida State Senate. In that race, he would challenge Sen. James E. King, Jr., who helped block the Florida Legislature's final efforts to force reinsertion of the PEG tube.

JUNE 27, 2005

Prosecutors find no evidence of wrongdoing by Michael Schiavo after Ms. Schiavo's collapse in 1990. They write: "If the available facts are analyzed without preconceptions, it is clear that there is no basis for further investigation. While some questions may remain following the autopsy, the likelihood of finding evidence that criminal acts were responsible for her collapse is not one of them....We strongly recommend that the inquiry be closed and no further action be taken."

JULY 7, 2005

Gov. Bush agrees to drop any further investigation into why Ms. Schiavo collapsed in 1990.

JULY 8, 2005

According to The Associated Press, "The fledgling Ave Maria University [in Naples, Florida] has established a scholarship in the name of Terri Schiavo for students planning careers in the priesthood."

AUGUST 5, 2005

The Florida State Guardianship Association names Michael Schiavo its "Guardian of the Year."

AUGUST 10, 2005

The New York Times reports that Senator Ron Wyden (D-Ore.) referred to Ms. Schiavo's case during a pre-confirmation-hearing meeting with President Bush's U.S. Supreme Court nominee, Judge John Roberts. Senator Wyden reportedly asked Judge Roberts whether he believed Congress should have taken the action it took. Although Judge Roberts reportedly refused to discuss the Schiavo case specifically, Senator Wyden recounts the judge's reply to a more general question as follows: "I am concerned with judicial independence. Congress can prescribe standards but when Congress starts to act like a court and prescribe particular remedies in particular cases, Congress has overstepped its bounds."

AUGUST 11, 2005

The New York Times reports that the White House disagrees with Senator Wyden's account. "Ed Gillespie, the chief White House lobbyist for Judge Roberts's Senate confirmation, sent a letter . . . saying that the notes taken by a White House aide during the session reflected a different response: `I am aware of court precedents which say Congress can overstep when it prescribes particular outcomes in particular cases.' " Senator Wyden stands by his earlier statement.

AUGUST 16, 2005

A conservative Catholic group wants 18 academics purged from campus for perpetuating "a culture of death" by backing abortion rights or siding against Terri Schiavo's parents, The Associated Press reports.

OCTOBER 18, 2005

A state judicial nominating commission announces that the lawyer who headed the DCF efforts to intervene in the Schiavo case is a finalist for two new state judgeships.

DECEMBER 7, 2005

Michael Schiavo establishes a political action committee—TerriPAC—to support or oppose politicians based on their positions regarding "government intrusion" in private lives. The "www.TerriPAC.org" site is no longer active.

JANUARY 21, 2006

Michael Schiavo marries his long-time girlfriend in a private ceremony in a church in Safety Harbor, some 15 miles northwest of Tampa.

FEBRUARY 12, 2006

Florida Senator Mel Martinez says that he may have been off-base in encouraging and voting for federal intervention in the Terri Schiavo matter. "Perhaps this was not in the realm of federal concern. It may have been better left to state courts to deal with it," Martinez said in a taped interview for Political Connections on Bay News 9.

MARCH 27, 2006

Just shy of one year after Ms. Schiavo's death, Michael Schiavo and professional writer Michael Hirsch publish a book titled *Terri: The Truth.*
At about the same time (just before the first anniversary of her death), Bob and Mary Schindler also publish a book, *A Life that Matters: The Legacy of Terri Schiavo.*

SEPTEMBER 5, 2006

Incumbent Florida Senator Jim King (R-Jacksonville) defeats anti-abortion activist Randall Terry in Terry's primary election bid sparked by the politics surrounding Ms. Schiavo's death.

MARCH 21, 2007

Terri Schiavo's brother, Bobby Schindler, writes a column criticizing presidential candidate and former Massachusetts Governor Mitt Romney for stating, "My view was a case like this [Schiavo] would normally be left in the hands of a court." According to Schindler, Romney was referring to and criticizing the attempt by Congress to help save Ms. Schiavo's life.

Schindler opines that this statement "could not be more wrong, morally or politically." He also speaks out against newspaper editors who won't publish his letters and praises the work of the Terri Schindler-Schiavo Foundation. He criticizes what he characterizes as a media bias in favor of Michael Schiavo, "no matter how patently suspicious his motives and character." The column appears in WorldNetDaily.com, a conservative website whose mission includes "revitalizing the role of the free press as a guardian of liberty."

APRIL 26, 2007

The Schiavo case appears in the 2008 presidential campaign when Sen. Barack Obama said during a debate that "he regretted not fighting Republican-led efforts in March 2005 to reconnect Ms. Schiavo's feeding tube," according to a *Miami Herald* report on an MSNBC interview. "'A lot of us, including me, left the Senate with a bill that allowed Congress to intrude where it shouldn't have,'" he said. (See also the entry for February 26, 2008.)

MAY 27, 2007

USA TODAY releases a list, "Lives of indelible impact," of 25 people "who moved us in the past quarter-century. Most are famous, but some are ordinary folks in extraordinary situations. Many became accidental leaders, even heroes, whose spirit enriched our lives." Ms Schiavo is No. 12 on the list, following Mother Teresa and Oprah Winfrey and preceding Michael J. Fox and Arthur Ashe.

SUMMER 2007

TerriPAC, the political action committee Michael Schiavo created, pays a $1,350 fine to the Federal Election Commission after failing to file complete and timely reports.

SEPTEMBER 14, 2007

The Vatican's "Congregation for the Doctrine of the Faith" issues a statement saying it is immoral to remove artificial hydration and nutrition from people in permanent vegetative states. The statement ("Responses to certain questions of the United States Conference of Catholic Bishops concerning artificial nutrition and hydration") is said to have been approved by Pope Benedict. U.S. bishops sought responses to questions about artificial hydration and nutrition in July 2005, shortly after the death of Ms. Schiavo.

NOVEMBER 18, 2007

Republican presidential candidate Fred Thompson says Ms. Schiavo should have been kept alive.

DECEMBER 11, 2007

The Terri Schindler Schiavo Foundation and Priests for Life jointly announce the establishment of an "International Day of Prayer and Remembrance for Terri Schindler Schiavo, and All of Our Vulnerable Brothers and Sisters" ("Terri's Day"), to be observed each year on March 31, the date of her death.

JANUARY 20, 2008

Judge Greer transfers from probate/guardianship court to family court, moving from judging guardianship cases to judging divorce cases.

FEBRUARY 26, 2008

During a presidential primary debate with Sen. Hillary Clinton, then-Sen. Barack Obama responds as follows to moderator Tim Russert's request to identify a statement or vote he'd like to take back: "Well, you know, when I first arrived in the Senate that first year, we had a situation surrounding Terri Schiavo. And I remember how we adjourned with a unanimous agreement that eventually allowed Congress to interject itself into that decisionmaking process of the families. It wasn't something I was comfortable with, but it was not something that I stood on the floor and stopped. And I think that was a mistake, and I think the American people understood that that was a mistake. And as a constitutional law professor, I knew better."

APRIL 30, 2008

The nine Republican state senators who played key roles in defeating proposed legislation in the Schiavo case in 2005 mostly stick together in voting down a bill that would have required women to undergo ultrasounds and review the results before obtaining abortions. Of the "Schiavo Nine," only Sen. J.D. Alexander of Lake Wales voted for this legislation. Nancy Argenziano is no longer in the Senate. The rest of the Schiavo Nine, who became known as "The Ultrasound Seven," are Lisa Carlton, Osprey; Mike Bennett, Bradenton; Paula Dockery, Lakeland; Evelyn Lynn, Ormond Beach; Dennis Jones, Seminole; Jim King, Jacksonville; and Burt Saunders, Naples.

Christopher Buckley, son of conservative writer and thinker William F. Buckley, who founded *The National Review*, resigns from his position with the magazine, stating, "While I regret this development, I am not in mourning, for I no longer have any clear idea what, exactly, the modern conservative movement stands for. Eight years of `conservative' government has brought us a doubled national debt, ruinous expansion of entitlement programs, bridges to nowhere, poster boy Jack Abramoff and an ill-premised, ill-waged war conducted by politicians of breathtaking arrogance. As a sideshow, it brought us a truly obscene attempt at federal intervention in the Terry *[sic]* Schiavo case."

Index ⠿

Abortion, 3, 19, 41, 203, 205, 209*n*.51. *See also* Fetus, *Roe v. Wade*
Advance directives, 1, 9, 50, 60, 91–92, 95, 102–109, 129, 197–199, 222
Allison, Dorothy, 150
American Academy of Neurology, 121, 129
American Association of People with Disabilities, 84
American Association on Mental Retardation, 17
American Medical Association, 208*n*.41
American Catholic Lawyers Association, 84
Anderson, Pat, 42
Aquinas, 7
Aristotle, 7
Artificial hydration and nutrition, 7, 10–11, 18, 26, 41, 79, 80, 86, 91, 93–97, 112, 158. *See also* PEG tube
Ashcroft, John, 14
Autonomy, 63, 65, 66, 101–109, 152, 181
Autopsy, *see* Schiavo, Terri, Autopsy

Bambakidis, Peter, 117, 119
Barnhill, James, 114
Batavia, Andrew, 181
Batza & Associates, 123
Beauchamp, Tom, 109
Belling, Catherine, 145
Benson, Steve, 16
Berger, Peter, 138

Best interests, 40, 48, 62–68, 82, 103. *See also* Substituted judgment
Bible, 104, 129, 141, 145. *See also* Koran
Bioethics, 29, 50, 63, 66, 101–103, 138–140, 149–150, 152–156
    National bioethicists' *amicus* brief, 63, 65
Blackstone, William, 67
Boorstin, Daniel, 212
Brain death, 24, 60–61, 155
Brain Injury Association of America, 208*n*.41
Brandeis, Louis, 53
Bresnahan, James, 147
Brophy, Paul, 124, 196
Browning, In re Guardianship of 60, 65, 79, 117, 208*n*.31
Busalacchi, Christine, 125
Bush, Jeb, 3, 14, 15, 39, 63, 69, 71, 72, 85–86, 89, 202
Bush, George W., 14, 24, 37*n*.41, 43–44, 47, 104
Byock, Ira, 153

California Medical Association, 107
Callahan, Daniel, 63, 74
Cantor, Norman, 91
Caplan, Art, 220
Catholic Church, 94–95, 146–147, 191
    International Congress on Life-Sustaining Treatments and Vegetative State: Scientific Advances and Ethical Dilemmas, 94

Catholic Medical Associations, World
    Federation of, 27, 208n.44
Center for Bioethics and Culture, 128
Chancery courts, 68
Cheshire, William, 123, 128
Childress, Jim, 109
Christian Medical and Dental
    Associations, 104, 106, 109, 128
Colby, William, 14
Coleman, Diane, 166, 169–170, 171, 179, 180
Coma, 145
Competence, 58–62, 91
Common law, 67
Consciousness, 7
Cooley, Thomas, 52–53
Cranford, Ron, vi, 121, 174
    Examination of Ms. Schiavo, 115–116
Creationism, 3, 4, 14
Cruzan, Nancy, 14, 16, 40, 54, 56–57, 93,
    125, 142, 145, 151, 196–197
*Cruzan v. Director, Missouri Dept. of
    Health*, 94, 95, 102
CT scans, 116, 171, 172
Culture Wars, 2, 8, 22, 28

Dehydration, 41, 63, 124–125. *See also*
    Starvation
Descartes, 7
Dialysis, 6
Didion, Joan, 141,197
Disability, 16–22, 87, 100n.32, 158–185
    "Ableism," 162
    Americans with Disability Act, 181
    Definition of, 16–17, 161–170
    Developmental, 182, 190n.84
    Disability rights, 4, 19–20, 81, 84–6,
        147, 153, 159–163, 166–170, 178–184,
        199–202
    Ideologies of normalcy, difference,
        160
Disability Rights Education and
    Defense Fund, 84
Drake, Steven, 201
Dresser, Rebecca, 106

Easter, 137, 141
Edwards, John, 127
Eisenberg, Jon, 13
Electroencephalogram (EEG), 116, 172
End-of-life care and decision making, 6,
    40, 61–62, 78, 82, 98

End-stage condition, 80
Ethics, 8, 10, 12, 51. *See also* Bioethics
Ethics committees, 1, 43, 148
Euthanasia, active, 3, 19. *See also* Suicide,
    ssisted

Feeding tubes, *see* PEG tubes
Felos, George, 62, 75n.28, 114, 121
Fetus, 7, 203–204, 209n.48–50. *See also*
    Abortion, *Roe v. Wade*
Fiore, Robin N., 7
Fletcher, John, 149
Flieshacker, Sam, 156
Florida, 5–6
    Flag, 5
Florida Bioethics Leaders' Analysis of
    HB 701, 124, 164, 208n.33
Florida Bioethics Network, vi
Florida Constitution, 70–71, 74, 79–80, 200
Florida Department of Children and
    Families, 72
Florida District Court of Appeal, 82–83,
    117, 119, 173, 177, 221
Florida Legislature, 19, 20, 21, 39, 40, 43,
    71, 79, 86, 87, 93, 95, 96, 102, 124
Florida Statutes, 66
Florida Supreme Court, 63, 79, 80, 82, 88,
    89, 93, 117, 200
Focus on the Family, 109
Fox News, 4, 214
Framing
    Disability rights, 199–202
    Fetal protection, 203–204
    Gender, 194–199
    Theory, 192–194
Frist, Bill, 126, 217, 220
Fuhrman, Mark, 3
Functional magnetic resonance imag-
    ing (fMRI), 32n.2, 127–128
Futility, 138

Gallagher, Hugh, 180
Gambone, Vincent, 117, 171
Gender. *See also* Women
    Gender essentialism, 192
    Frame, 194–199
    Norms, 195, 205
    Stereotypes, 191,195–197
Genetic testing, 20
Gibbs, David, 123
Gibson, Mel, 35n.27

God, 10, 143, 35*n*.23, 104, 141, 143, 172
Golenski, John, 146
Grace, Nancy, 141
Greer, George, 3, 32*n*.10, 39, 51, 59, 61, 62, 67, 72, 81, 98, 103, 114, 117, 118, 122, 128, 129, 170, 173, 177
Greer, Melvin, 117, 121
Griswold v. Connecticut, 52, 75*n*.5
Guardianship, 50, 62–68, 88–90, 114

Half the Planet Foundation, 84
Hammesfahr, William, 117–119, 122, 125, 131, 174
Hannity, Sean, 4
Hastings Center, 63, 109*n*.5
Hastings Center Guidelines on the Termination of Life Sustaining Treatment and the Care of the Dying, 63, 64, 109*n*.5
Hentoff, Nat, 38*n*.44
Holmes, Oliver Wendell, 53–54
Hospice, 1, 19
Hospice Patients' Alliance, 84
Hyperbaric oxygen therapy, 118, 174

Informed consent. *See* Valid consent and refusal
International Task Force on Euthanasia and Assisted Suicide, 84
Islamic religious law, 155
Israel, 145
Italian National Committee on Bioethics, 97

Jackson Jesse, 35*n*.27, 217
Jewish religious law, 147
John F. Kennedy Memorial Hospital v. Bludworth, 117
Journalism, *See* News media
Judicial activism, 2, 4, 14, 22–23, 36*n*.36
Justinian, 67

Kant, Immanuel, 7–8, 10, 34*n*.17
King, Florida Senator Jim, 15
Koch, Tom, 160–162
Koran, 145. *See also* Bible

Language, 23–27, 72–73. *See also* Semantics
Lapertosa, Max, 201
Last Acts, 208*n*.41
Living wills. *See* Advance directives

Lebensunwerten Lebens, 20
Levinas, Emmanuel, 154, 155
Lochner v. New York, 53
Locke, 7, 57–68
Louisiana, 68

MacNeil, Robert, 212
Malpractice, 12, 47
Marbury v. Madison, 55
Martinez, Mel, 16
Maryland, 198
Maxfield, William, 117–119, 174
Mayo Clinic, 129
McCormick, Richard, 146
Medicaid, 5, 45, 47
Medical examiner, 51, 129–130. *See also* Schiavo, Terri, Autopsy; Thogmartin, Jon
Meilaender, Gilbert, 106
Miller, Robert, 46
Minimally conscious state, 51, 86
Missouri, 55–56, 196
Murrow, Edward R., 222

National Council on Independent Living, 84
National Right to Life Committee Model Legislation, 100*n*.44
National Spinal Cord Injury Association, 84
Nazis, 20, 21, 180–181, 202
Nelson, Stephen J., 128, 129, 130
Neurology, 26, 58–59, 114–116, 118, 131–132, 173. *See also* PVS
News media, 10, 23, 41, 89, 139–140, 142, 143–144, 210–222
    Bias of open questions, 217–219
    Bias of objectivity, 214–216
    Bias of perceived credibility, 216–217
    Bias of visual emphasis, 219–221
    Philosophical issues, grappling with, 217, 219
    Public journalism, 215
    Political pressure, source of, 211
    Television news, mandates of, 212–214
    Unprepared reporters, 219
New York, 68
Nilsson, Lennart, 203
Not Dead Yet, 36*n*.31, 84, 153, 171, 178, 201, 208*n*.41

Operation Rescue. *See* Terry, Randall
Oregon, 169

Paris, John, 146, 147
Parkinson's Action Network, 208*n*.42
Passover, 137, 141
Paternalism, 106–108
Patient Self Determination Act, 147
PEG tube, 2, 6, 11–12, 19, 25–26, 81–85,
    87. *See also* Artificial hydration and
    nutrition
PET scan, 127
Percutaneous endoscopic gastrostomy.
    See PEG tube
Perlman, Itzhak, 168
Permanent vegetative state. *See* PVS
Persistent vegetative state. *See* PVS
Personhood, 7–9, 33*n*.11, 74
Peterson, Laci, 141
Plato, 7
Politics,18–20, 39, 41, 45, 67, 98, 184–185
Pontifical Academy for Life Congress,
    27, 208*n*.44
Pope John Paul II, 27, 39, 94–95, 145, 146,
    217
President's Council on Bioethics,
    104–106, 109, 146
Priests for Life, 104, 109
Principlism, 109*n*.5
Privacy, 40, 52–57, 71, 75*n*.5, 79, 120, 137,
    217
Professionals for Excellence in Health
    Care, 84
PVS, 2, 6, 7–10, 27, 31*n*.1, 50–51, 61, 75*n*.2,
    79, 80, 81, 85, 93, 99*n*.7, 112–121,
    123, 129–130, 145, 170–171. *See also*
    Neurology

Quinlan, Karen Ann, 39, 51, 59, 60–61,
    75*n*.3–4, 93, 139, 142, 144, 145, 148,
    195–196, 220

Rationality, 7–9
Ravitsky, Vardit, 157*n*.14
Reeve, Christopher, 127
    Paralysis Foundation, 208*n*.42
Rehnquist, William, 55, 57
Relativism, 46
Religion, 144–148
Resource allocation, 40, 43–44
    Treatment requests, refusals, 9, 20,
    82, 200

Robert Wood Johnson Foundation, 3, 61,
    208*n*.41
Roe v. Wade, 74. *See also* Abortion

Scalia, Antonin, 54, 56
Schiavo I, 81–83, 89, 92
Schiavo II, 81–83
Schiavo III, 83–85
Schiavo IV, 85
Schiavo, Michael, 2, 3, 12, 16, 25, 39,
    46, 51, 57, 60, 66, 73, 74, 80, 83, 87,
    114–115, 140, 171, 178, 197
    As guardian, 10, 12
Schindler, Robert and Mary, 2, 12, 41, 43,
    46, 78, 80, 83, 87, 112, 122, 145, 173, 204
Schiavo, Terri,
    Autopsy, 2, 51, 125, 129–130, 133, 133.
        See also Medical examiner
    Cardiac arrest, 114, 163
    Cause célèbre, as, 16–17, 41–41
    Death of, 16, 101
    Oral advance directive, 117, 219
    PVS diagnosis, 115–116, 118, 218–219
    Subpoenaed by U.S. House of
        Representatives, 16
    Videos of, 2, 32*n*.10, 116, 121–122, 211,
        218, 220
Schwartz, Peter, 26
Self-Advocates Becoming Empowered,
    84
Semantics, 31*n*.1, 77*n*.49, 219
Silvers, Anita, 181
Simpson, O.J., 3, 221
Sleeping Beauty, 194–195
Soul, 6, 46
Starvation, 26, 63, 97, 124–125. *See also*
    Dehydration
Starvation and Dehydration of Persons
    with Disabilities Prevention Act,
    86, 95, 124, 199
Steinberg commission, 147
Stem cell research, 3, 4, 14, 34*n*.15, 127
Substituted judgment, 40, 62, 66, 92–93,
    103, 199, 200. *See also* Best interests
Suicide, 7
    Assisted, 11–12, 19, 45
Surrogates and proxies, 11, 12, 21, 80, 82,
    87–91, 103, 105, 179, 198

Technology, medical, 6, 8, 46, 147, 152–153
Television, 45. *See also* News media

Terminal condition, 80
Terri's Law, 5, 19, 36*n*.32, 40, 69–73, 86–89, 97, 98, 175
Terri Schindler Schiavo Foundation, 14, 125
Terry, Randall, 14–15, 35*n*.27, 217
Texas, 47
Thalamic stimulator, 128, 176
Thogmartin, Jon, 125, 129–130. *See also* Autopsy, Medical examiner
Timeline of Key Events in the Case of Theresa Marie Schiavo, v-vi
Treatise of the Law of Torts, 52
Tyler, Beverly, 61–61

Union Pacific Railway Co. v. Botsford, 102
Utilitarianism, 11
U.S. Constitution, 52–55, 65, 68–69
U.S. Food and Drug Administration, 128
U.S. House of Representatives, 16
U.S. presidential campaigns, 4, 126, 251
U.S. Senate, 15
U.S. Supreme Court, 94, 95, 96, 102

Valid consent and refusal, 21, 33*n*.13
Vasodilation therapy, 118, 174
Vegetative state. *See* PVS

Velasco, Raul de, 34*n*.18–19
Ventilators, 6, 51
Vitalism, 2, 19, 86, 91

Warren, Charles, 53
Washington v. Harper, 77*n*.50
Webber, Fred, 117, 120, 173
Weldon, Dave, 126
Weller, Barbara, 33*n*.10
Wendland, Robert, 142, 145, 208*n*.41
Wilson, James, 54–55
Wolf, Susan, 197
Wolfson, Jay, 13, 125
    As guardian *ad litem*, 39–40
    Interactions with Ms. Schiavo, 43
    Report to governor, 13, 40, 45, 47–48, 175–176, 202
Women. *See also* Gender
    Caregiving, 204–205
    End of life, 195–196
    Moral agency, 204–205
World Association of Persons with Disabilities, 85
World Health Organization, 163, 164
World Institute on Disability, 85
World Wide Web, v, 48

Zabeiga, Thomas, 123

CPSIA information can be obtained at www.ICGtesting.com
Printed in the USA
237300LV00001B/6/P